Psychoana[...]
Theory, Therapy,
and the Self

PSYCHOANALYTIC THEORY, THERAPY, AND THE SELF

A Basic Guide to the Human Personality
in Freud, Erikson, Klein,
Sullivan, Fairbairn, Hartmann,
Jacobson, and Winnicott

HARRY GUNTRIP, Ph. D.

Fellow, British Psychological Society,
Psychotherapist and Lecturer, Leeds University
Department of Psychiatry

Basic Books, Inc., Publishers · *New York*

FOREWORD

===

In 1968 Dr. Harry Guntrip visited the William Alanson White Institute of Psychiatry, Psychoanalysis, and Psychology, as Visiting Distinguished Psychoanalyst. This volume is the written record of two seminars—one on theory, the other on clinical material. The unwritten record is much larger and perhaps more significant than the written. Dr. Guntrip brought a zest, a warmth, and a sparkling humor to his material, both theoretical and clinical. His intense interest, his patience, and his serious caring enlivened and stimulated a whole group of people to think more clearly about their ideas and their way of practicing.

"To care for people," writes Guntrip, "is more important than to care for ideas." This humane attitude is evidenced throughout in Harry Guntrip's approach to his patients, to his colleagues, and to theorists both past and present. First and foremost, he feels the experience with the patient, and from the experience, he conceptualizes so that theory is very close to experience. Though Guntrip is most clearly associated with Fairbairn and Winnicott, he is not identified with any school. This independence of thought leads to a very concise exposition and critique of Freud, Sullivan, Klein, Erikson, Fairbairn, Hartmann, Jacobson and Winnicott. "I came to the conclusion," he says, "that particularly, theories about human nature always represent a modicum of fact described within the limits of the cultural outlook of some one restricted period of social history." Dr. Guntrip's emphasis is on the essential quality of personal life, not on the machinery. He explores in some detail his reasons for believing that analysis should include a regression beyond the limits called for by the classical Freudian school. This is to facilitate the patient's regression beyond the Oedipal to the pre-genital stages. Being accepted and understood in the schizoid position enables the patient to feel hopeful and to be "born again." Whatever the merits or the practicality of this approach, Dr. Guntrip makes a persuasive humane case.

The White Institute is pleased to have this record published.

EARL G. WITENBERG

PREFACE TO THE 1973
Basic Books Paperback
EDITION

≡

The undisputed starting-point of the modern psychodynamic study of the human personality is the work of Sigmund Freud from the late 1880s to 1938. It is fashionable for some intellectuals, still steeped in nineteenth-century positivism and empiricism, to decry Freud as unscientific. In fact there are two aspects of his work, the theory (based on his own nineteenth-century positivist scientific education) and the acute clinical factual observations he made of actual psychopathological phenomena. The theory, like that of all great scientists grows dated, the clinical facts remain to be extended. Dr. R. Harré (Oxford) writes: "Freud was a great scientist because he looked for the causes of such commonplace occurrences as slips of the tongue, as well as for the causes of such unusual happenings as fits of hysteria" (*The Philosophies of Science, Oxford*, p. 115). Critics of the scientific status of psychoanalysis must take account of the tremendous changes that have come about in the philosophy of science, in the post-Einstein, post-positivist era. Harré sums this up: "Positivism restricts empirical knowledge to the passing show of sense-experience. . . . The realist point of view emphasizes the work of human imagination in leading to conceptions of the realities behind experience. I believe the case against positivism on intellectual, historical and moral grounds to be overwhelming." (op. cit., Preface.) Freud the positivist by education, was constantly being left behind unwittingly by Freud the realist face to face with suffering patients. As a result, psychoanalysis, the systematic, i.e. scientific, study of psychodynamic phenomena in the only possible laboratory, the clinical personal relationship, has gone on steadily and progressively changing. There has been an interaction of inquiring minds on a worldwide scale, many of them outside the narrowly organized psychoanalytic movement. It would not be either good or possible for psychodynamic research to be confined to a few closed schools of theory. In addition to the original Freudian, Adlerian and Jungian Societies, America now has its "American Academy of Psychoanalysis" with its own journal, and the "Journal of Contemporary Psychoanalysis" of the W. A. White Institute, New York. In Britain, the newly formed Royal College of Psychiatrists has a special "Psychotherapy Section" which must inevitably foster research in this field.

In a book of this size it is impossible to mention the contributions of many of even the most important workers. I have omitted Jung, although Freudians and Jungians in Britain have made some attempts to find common ground. I have also omitted Adler, though he recognized the fundamental importance of the Ego or Personal Self long before Freud did. Official psychoanalysis only moved beyond the "biological Id" to the truly "psychological Ego," after the First World War, in Freud's monographs of the 1920s. My aim has been narrower, and is indicated by the few names in the chapter headings. I think they will not be questioned as representing predominantly the particular lines of development I have chosen to trace.

The material presented in this small book is the substance of a series of lectures I gave at The William Alanson White Institute of Psychiatry, Psychoanalysis and Psychology in New York, and The Washington School of Psychiatry. Some of it was presented on brief visits to the Austen Riggs Center, Stockbridge, and the Adult Psychiatry Section of the Department of Mental Health, in the Bethesda National Institute of Health. The basis of Chapters 2 to 5 is four lectures on "Object-Relations Theory" or "Interpersonal Relations Theory." Chapters 6 and 7 abbreviate a series of seminars on "Treatment of Schizoid Persons." Much of this material was also elaborated on a visit to the Los Angeles Psychoanalytic Society in 1969. I have been urged by a number of people to write a condensed account of the over-all theoretical position set forth in my larger research books.[1] I hope this small volume will serve exactly that purpose, and will be found useful to students in particular, with whom pressure on time seldom permits the study of many larger volumes. On the other hand this skeleton of theory may well prepare the way for the exploration of larger books, where the intellectual bare bones of theory are clothed with the flesh and blood of actual clinical material; concepts are related closely to the evidence that called for their formulation; and where wider aspects of Winnicott's work are dealt with.

I welcome the opportunity here provided to take into account the work of Jacobson, and were I writing the book now de novo I would certainly devote a section to Balint's book *The Basic Fault* with its extremely valuable exposition of the patient's need to "regress," not in search of "satisfactions" of so-called instinctive needs, but rather in search of "Recognition" as a "Person." This adds a highly important emphasis to Fairbairn's view that "the Ego in Personal Relationships" is the key psychodynamic concept, and Winnicott's stress on the growth of "basic Ego-relatedness" in the baby, in the primary mother-infant relation. I have mentioned only very briefly, the changes in outlook in the philosophy of science, in general psychology, and in biology, that have taken place since Freud began his work. I would like to add here a brief reference to one very important view in epistemology, for psychoanalysis. Scientists have so often drawn the distinction between "external reality" as capable of objective scientific investigation, and "internal, subjective experience" as not amenable to objective study. Only "objective phenomena" are then spoken of as "real." Subjective phenomena are dismissed as fantasy. That distinction is clearly itself unreal. Our subjective experiences are "subjective to ourselves" and are also in inescapable ways "objectively real to other people." If someone threatens us, we must know whether he *really* means it. Hitler's megalomaniac delusions, and Stalin's paranoid delusions had terrible objective reality for everyone. Only intellectual prejudice can dismiss "subjective reality" as mere fantasy. It is the very stuff of our living, the "psychodynamic phenomena" psychoanalysis must study. Contemporary philosophy of science and epistemology make this possible. "The hierarchical model of the structure of knowledge" describes "reality" as existing on a series of different levels, like floors of a building; with physics and chemistry on the bottom floor, and rising floor by floor above them, the progressive complexities of inorganic, organic, social and psychological phenomena. At each level, as Medawar puts it, "New ideas seem to emerge which are inexplicable in the language or with the conceptual resources of the tier below. We cannot interpret sociology in terms of biology, or biology in terms of physics." (*Induction and Intuition in Scientific Thought*, Jayne Lectures, The American Philosophical Society, 1968.) We must add that neither can we interpret psychology in terms of biology, neurophysiology, or any lower level science. Reductionism and its Behaviorist extremes are out of date.

Finally I take the opportunity of this edition to add a further word about Fairbairn's theoretical description of endopsychic structure (p. 98). Any theory of endopsychic structure is a kind of "conceptual map" of the diverse aspects or provinces of our disintegrated psychic functioning: useful provided we do not regard them as entities with rigid boundaries, on the "spatial" implications of such a term as "Ego-splitting." They are simultaneous ways of fluid emotional functioning of one and the same psychic self, even though they are mutually conflicting. The processes of "repression" create the illusion of "boundaries." The theoretical labels are guides to what to look for, and the analysis is always open to revision in the light of clinical experience. There is at present some confusion in conceptualizing the deepest or earliest "splits" in the psychic Self or Person-Ego. Fairbairn's analysis of Ego-splitting as a result of bad-object experience, only went as deep as the identification of the Libidinal Ego (L. E.), the infant's basic nature in a state of needing mother. He wrote to me that he could not fit Regression into that scheme, and accepted my suggestion of a final Ego-split. A L. E. goes on clamoring for mother to meet its needs, while another part loses hope, gives up, becomes an apathetic Regressed Ego (Rd. E.), the basis of the worst depersonalized schizoid experience. Winnicott wrote to ask me "Is your Rd. E. withdrawn or repressed?" In fact it becomes both. At first it is withdrawn, falling back into apathy, its potentialities for growth unevoked by the mother's failure to relate to her baby. But then it must become repressed, lest its eruption should cause a conscious state of depersonalization. Fairbairn could not account for this experience because he regarded the infant as "a pristine whole Ego at birth." Winnicott was content to say "the baby is a whole human being at birth," and "the self at this very early stage is only potential." If the mother fails the baby, he regards its "true self as put into cold storage awaiting a chance of rebirth into a better environment." I would say that the infant is "a whole psyche with human ego-potential at birth" and it depends on the mother's "relating," whether this potential is evoked and grows a real Ego or Personal Self. If not, the "true self" is not so much "put back into cold storage" but left unevoked by lack of any object-relationship in which it could grow. This is a matter of degree and artificial false selves are developed on a conscious level as substitutes. In that deepest split-off bit of the psyche, which includes experiences of being unevoked, withdrawn and repressed, lie the sources of the worst schizoid and schizophrenic states. The therapist's supreme obligation to the patient is to supply that element of "relating" which Balint called "Recognition."

Finally I would express on behalf of my wife and myself, our deep appreciation of the warm hospitality we everywhere received, and of the invigorating keenness of discussion following every lecture. The world needs not just a theory of personal relationships, but evidence that it is possible to practice it in working together in this and other fields. I must also thank Basic Books for their helpfulness at every stage from manuscript to publication, when geographical distance made personal contacts impossible.

NOTE

1. Harry Guntrip, *Personality Structure and Human Interaction,* The International Psycho-Analytical Library (London: The Hogarth Press; New York: International Universities Press, 1961); *Schizoid Phenomena, Object-Relations and the Self,* The International Psycho-Analytical Library (London: The Hogarth Press; New York: International Universities Press, 1968); "The Object-Relations Theory of W. R. D. Fairbairn," *The American Handbook of Psychiatry,* vol. 1 (New York: Basic Books, 1973), chap. 39.

CONTENTS

═══

PART I
Theory

PART II
Therapy

PART

I

Theory

Chapter 1

SEEING FREUD
IN PERSPECTIVE

===

Quoting Freud in psychoanalysis is beginning at last to be like quoting Newton in physics. Both men are assured of that permanent place in the history of thought that belongs to the genuine pioneer. It is not the function of the pioneer to say the last word but to say the first word. That is the most difficult step. All the pioneer has to begin with is a problem, which has always been there, but hitherto no one has looked at that phenomenon in this particular way. The pioneer suddenly asks a new kind of question. Once the all-important start has been made along some new line of investigation, those who come after have only to faithfully follow up every possible line of inquiry it suggests. Some of these will be false trails, others will lead somewhere, but all have to be explored.

Freud started on the path of the pioneer when, because of the necessity to earn a living, he turned from his laboratory to clinical work. No doubt he was not the first neurologist to feel skeptical about the efficacy of the cures of that era for neurotic symptoms, but no one else reacted as Freud did. The investigations of Charcot and the French hypnotists were certainly a help, but it was Freud's insight that led him to cast hypnosis aside and begin to formulate the creative idea that the symptoms of neurosis had a meaning that could be explained in terms of the patient's life history. Hitherto medical symptoms had been simply cold physical facts (which most of them still are), but Freud found that some were different. Some psychoneuroses involve physical symptoms that are connected more with the patient's personal relationships in family life, than with biochemistry or organic disease. Freud found that at least with hysteric neuroses the symptoms could disappear when the patient felt secure with the physician, and reappear if that relationship was disturbed. Thus, slowly, a whole new area of facts began to come to light, not only concerning some types of physical symptom, but also concerning states of mind and modes of behavior.

This area of investigation has demanded intensive study ever since. But it is a striking fact that, at any rate in Britain, those who criticize psychoanalysis rarely show firsthand knowledge of events in the field later than the Freud of about 1908, when his paper on "Civilized Sexual Morality and Modern Nervousness" was written.

This presented in an uncompromising way the classic psychoanalytical "Instinct Theory" that all our troubles are due to the repression of instincts, and that since sublimation (or diverting instinctive energies to socially approved goals) is so hard, most of us are doomed to be either neurotic or criminal, that is, antisocial. Dr. Martin James describes how gradually Freud's early ideas came to influence progressive thinkers in education and child-rearing and

created confusion about Freud's ideas because of the paradox that the patron saint adopted for revolutionary propositions was Freud, and Freud was not consulted. He was a proper, conventional moral man and would have rejected much of what was done in his name. . . . The cathartic movement began early in the twentieth century and had the motto "no repressions," . . . the do-as-you-please school and the slogan of "Freedom." . . . The response of psychoanalysts to this state of affairs was to stress an opposite side of the story. . . . They have over the last twenty years been at pains to explain the *need* for repression and that symptom-formation is even the sign of a strong ego.[1]

This premature attempt to make popular use of Freud's new work seems to have had the result of fixating the meaning of psychoanalysis in the general mind as standing only for Freud's early views. Thus, a Cambridge psychologist, Dr. Max Hammerton, writes:

I am an experimental psychologist. . . . but most of the people I meet seem to imagine that my stock in trade consists of a couch and a lot of verbiage about libido and id and what not. Sometimes I heartily wish that Dr. Freud had never been born.[2]

Dr. Hammerton and many similar critics, of whom the behaviorist psychologists have been the most vocal, show little sign of being acquainted at firsthand with the far-reaching changes that have occurred in psychoanalytic theory and practice since Freud's early days.

Today the question to ask is not so much "What did Freud say?" but "What has Freud's work led on to?" It is all that Freud started that becomes increasingly important. Psychoanalysis can no longer be simply identified with the original, classic psychobiology. Freud himself began the first major move beyond that starting point, when in the 1920s he turned his attention to the analysis of the "ego." A Professor of Psychiatry whose interests are mainly biochemical once said to me "Freud is the easiest writer to make contradict himself." In fact this was a tribute to a fearless thinker whose mind was ever on the move, exploring the little understood ways of the human mind. He was a pioneer who opened up an entirely new field of systematic inquiry into the inner workings of human experience.

This field had traditionally been explored in literature, religion, and in the symbolism of art, but no one before Freud had attempted, in the particularly personal way that he did, a systematic examination of the emotional disturbances of human beings that find expression in mental illness, disturbed behavior, and so on. Such an infinitely complex inquiry could not possibly have been completed and exhausted by Freud; and where his work is now leading becomes ever more important than where it began. At this point it becomes important to draw a distinction between Freud's clinical experiences, the psychic phenomena with which he was confronted in his patients, and the theories he formulated to coordinate and, if possible, explain them. This distinction is not always easy to make, because psychic phenomena are not visible as tangible "things" obviously existing in relative isolation from other "things." They are subjective experiences which different people verbalize in different ways. Nevertheless, the description of certain common experiences by people of extremely different types are found to have a cumulative consistency. The psychoanalyst, being himself human, can recognize the meaning of what they say by reference to his own experience. Moreover, what is in this sense clinically observable is found to imply the existence of other subjective experiences which have to be inferred to make sense of what is more directly known. Thus, the unconscious is both a clinical fact and an inference, or hypothesis. To illustrate this point concretely, a male patient dreamed furiously every night but could remember nothing of it in the morning. So he took a pencil and paper up to bed to write the dreams down in the night, only to find that he did not dream. After four nights he concluded that he had ceased to dream and did not take up his pencil and paper. As before, he dreamed furiously and remembered nothing in the morning. The inference is inescapable that he was determined not to allow his dreams to become conscious (probably because his waking self was too afraid to know how disturbed he felt deep down and why), but he was quite unconscious of this determination, for all that it was a powerfully operative fact in his experience of himself. Having made this discovery, he did then begin slowly to remember some of his troubled dream-life. All this kind of experience that Freud steadily accumulated, I shall call the "clinical facts he discovered," and distinguish them from "the theories he formulated to explain them." Broadly, Freud's observations of matters of psychic fact have proved to be more lasting than his theories, even though we cannot draw an absolute distinction between them. In his theory making Freud was bound to be primarily influenced by his scientific education and by the ideas generally accepted in the cultural era in which he began his work. His factual discoveries were among the new influences that have led to further cultural change. This is how it is with all creative minds; their original work drives them beyond the boundaries of their own educational inheritance. What I have sought to do in this short series of lectures is to trace the changes that have gone on and are now going on, in psychoanalytical theory, from the starting point Freud provided as long ago as the 1890s.

I have stated that much of Freud's clinical observation of psychic experiences as verifiable matters of fact, turning up again and again in the widest variety of persons, has proved to be of permanent validity and importance. To illustrate this we can refer to such experiences as the various forms of fear and anxiety, love and sexual desire, anger, hate, jealousy and aggression, and the conflicts that ensue between these experiences when they occur, as they often do, simultaneously in the same person. We can also refer to evidence relating to the ways in which such conflicts often result in the repression of some of the conflicting emotions, which nevertheless do not thereby cease to be felt, but continue to be experienced albeit unconsciously, with highly disturbing effects on conscious experience and behavior. Out of this inwardly suppressed mental turbulence, there arise the various symptoms of psychoneurosis, both physical and mental. This disturbance is not confined to illness, but in some cases is acted out as antisocial or even criminal behavior. This repressed psychic experience finds yet a third outlet in dreams by night and in daydreams or fantasies by day. This type of psychic experience lends itself in a unique way to being understood as having meanings that are intelligible in terms of the person's life history. Dreams can even contain disguised or plain and undisguised memories of past traumatic events; but, furthermore, dreams are largely, if not entirely, a reliving during sleep of all the unresolved emotional problems in human relationships of our entire past life, if it has been a disturbed past. Thus if a person makes a dream the starting point for talking out a free flow of thought, he will steadily find that he is exploring anew all that he has been unable to deal with satisfactorily in the past, and that this buried, disturbed experience can and usually does, in time, lead back to surprisingly early childhood. It becomes apparent that we do not by any means entirely grow out of our childhood experiences, and that, in so far as they are a source of acute anxiety and insecurity and angers, a great deal of all this is buried in the unconscious while our conscious self of everyday living develops on either a conformity or a rebellion basis, or more usually a mixture of the two. Our conscious self has to develop ego-defences against the uprush of subtle intrusion of the turbulent unconscious conflicts. When these defences weaken or fail, the buried legacy of a too disturbed past erupts into consciousness to result in all degrees of mental or personal malfunctioning, ranging from mild anxiety symptoms to severe or, for the time being, total breakdown of adult mental functioning. All this inevitably puts great stress on the enormous importance of the formative experiences of early childhood. It was Freud who first acted on the assumption that prevention is better than cure for adults by treating a phobia of horses in a five-year-old boy, as long ago as 1909. Today child guidance clinics have proliferated everywhere.

Freud further discovered that one of the things that happens to repressed experiences in childhood is that later in life the emotions involved find an outlet by transference onto some roughly analogous figure in the present day. This phenomenon of "transference"—so prolific a cause of disruption in friendships, marriages, and adult partnerships of all kinds—inevitably erupts, unrecognized by the person in the treatment situation. The therapist, then, gets a chance to help the patient gradually to recognize and grow out of these survivals of past experience and to become free to relate in emotionally realistic and appropriate ways to people in the present day. Freud discovered that in the end, the main method of helping people to outgrow their buried emotional past and to free themselves for a new development of personality towards friendly, spontaneous, and creative living in the present, was simply to leave the person entirely free to talk out whatever occurred to him. This is not as easy as it sounds, for sooner or later it involves the free voicing of what has for a lifetime been held to be prohibited. But, slowly, as the patient finds that he does not lose the analyst's respect, and is taken entirely seriously, he is helped to understand and accept much that has always puzzled him about himself. Then, in spite of periods of severe strain, the over-all effect of this process is an increasing sense of liberation and reality in oneself. The patient begins to understand how human living, always dependent on the quality of the human relationships we have the good or bad fortune to encounter, can be recreated in the freeing and security-giving new relationship offered by the therapist. Reliability, sympathetic objectivity, and the genuine understanding offered by the analyst, enables the emotionally disturbed person slowly to acquire the confidence to "free associate," i.e., to talk his way freely out of the emotional mire of past unhappiness in which he has been bogged down. And this enables

9

him to make realistic and appropriate relationships with all the people, beginning with his therapist, with whom he must deal in his present day living. Among other things, he learns to recognize and not to rationalize his own motives and to understand other people better, because he now understands himself. All this and more could be cited as exemplifying the *factual clinical discoveries* made by Freud which hold good permanently, because they are recognizable human experiences, capable of being observed in all of us.

As an example of the more subtle and penetrating insightful discoveries made by Freud, I will give a single instance. Freud observed that "Identification is a substitute for a lost human relationship," or indeed for one that was urgently needed and unobtainable. Thus a child who finds that he cannot get any satisfactory kind of relationship with a parent who is too cold and aloof, or too aggressive, or too authoritarian tends to make up for his sense of apartness and isolation by identifying with, or growing like, that parent, as if this were a way of possessing the needed person within oneself. Freud's writings abound with such searching insights. It is this body of factual observation of human experience that constitutes the permanent contribution of Freud. It is this that theories seek to explain and systematize in a coherent body of synthesized understanding of human nature. Freud, naturally, made his own attempts at theoretical explanation, and here we have to say that though his theories, which he himself was always changing and developing, proved to be a most stimulating starting point, they were of necessity lacking in the permanence of his factual discoveries. All theories, especially those about human nature, are conditioned by the cultural era, the prevailing intellectual climate, and the dominant ideas of the time in which they are developed. Freud's theorizing was of necessity highly determined from the start by the scientific education in physics, chemistry, physiology, neurology, and general medicine and also by the prevailing ideas in academic psychology, philosophy, and social studies then prevalent. It was part of Freud's fate, which involved him in no little mental pain, that his own developing insights into human nature compelled him so often to clash with the legacy of his own educational heritage and the thinking of his contemporaries.

It is the far-reaching changes in theory construction since Freud began that I have endeavored to sketch, as clearly as possible, within the limited space of this small book. Few people, outside of those whose special professional concern it is to keep their data up-to-date, are aware how much the original theory has changed. Even the most important contributors are far too numerous for any but a small number of them to be mentioned and their work assessed here. I have chosen, therefore, to select what seemed to me the most important single line of central and consistent development and to illustrate that by dealing with the few leading psychodynamic thinkers most closely related to it.

This basic theme arises, as I see it, from a study of Freud's own work. Beginning as a highly trained physical science laboratory worker, Freud was slowly pushed by his experiences with patients beyond the physical into the study of the dynamically disturbed psychological, emotional, highly individual, and meaningful life of human beings as persons in their most important relationships with one another, beginning with that of the parent and child. People with otherwise healthy constitutions can become ill because of sheer distress in the basic relations of life. This fact was well known among family doctors, but Freud was the first to investigate it on a purely psychodynamic level. Here was his personal paradox. He was trained to be a physical scientist but was destined to become the creator of a new psychodynamic science. All through his work, two strands of thought were interwoven, the physical and the psychological, or personal. Very slowly the personalistic thinking emerged to the forefront, taking precedence over the physicalistic thinking.

It will suffice at this point to indicate the general nature of the shift that has evolved. At the beginning Freud sought to base all his explanations on physical factors. His first theory of "anxiety" was that it was dammed up sexual tension, denied any healthy outlet. Dr. Leo Rangell, in a lecture in London, stated that it took Freud twenty-five years, in spite of urging from Dr. Ernest Jones, to give up this physical theory for the psychological theory that anxiety is an ego-defense reaction to danger—a signal in one's self-experience of some imminent threat. Here we see the shift of emphasis from psychobiological instincts to the ego or self. Freud had sought to explain all human motivation by reference to two innate instincts, the drives of sex and aggression, but since the turn of the century the idea of instinct which was unquestioned in Freud's day has been carefully researched and proved to be a very unclear and unsatisfactory concept, by no means rehabilitated by the work of the ethologists. Sex is better regarded as an appetite; and aggression, not as an innate drive to hostile, attacking behavior, but, like anxiety, as an ego-reaction to threat, especially a threat to the personality. Freud's later psychological theory of anxiety indicates his major shift in theoretical emphasis, from instincts to the ego. He did not, however, abandon the "instinct theory," which hindered a full, realistic treatment of the ego as the personal self; he oscillated between treating it as a self and then again as a control-system which was only a part of the whole person. Much psychoanalytical discussion has raged around this question. I will only observe here that psychoanalytical theory today centers less and less on the control of instinct and more on the development of a stable core of selfhood—that is, the laying of the foundations of a strong personal ego in a good mother-infant relationship at the start of life, and its subsequent fate in the ever varying types of personal relationships, good and bad, that make up our life. The details of this change of theoretical emphasis will be worked out in the subsequent chapters by surveying the work of those leading thinkers who have played the most important roles in this development. Psychoanalysis threatened to come to a dead end if it remained tied to the instinct theory, but the truly psychological essence of it has emerged in the "Object-Relations Theory" (a term which is further illuminated by Harry Stack Sullivan's term "Interpersonal Relations Theory").

Psychoanalysis could derive much help, so far as theory-formulation is concerned, from general psychology, especially now that there are signs of revolt among psychologists against the rigid behaviorism of such writers as James Skinner and Hans Eysenck. As R. Phillips has stated, "To the unbiased observer the increasing dependence of experimental psychologists upon complex gadgetry is obviously yet another sign of man's alienation from his fellow man. . . . What we need is a great leap backwards to the psychology of our forefathers, when experimenter and subject faced each other in a warm friendly relationship." [3] Phillips regards the testing apparatus today as "erected by the experimenter as a sort of last ditch defence mechanism," and concludes, "Only the study of psychology can save us from this: that psychological psychology in which the proper study of mankind is subjects." [4] Psychoanalysis would have much in common with a truly personal human psychology of this kind. Another sign of the times is that an increasing number of physical scientists are being driven by the growth of their own physical specialities to casting serious doubts on the orthodox scientific materialism of Victorian and post-Victorian times. Dr. Jacob Bronowski, of The Salk Institute of Biology, holds that man is both a machine and a self, and that there are two qualitatively different kinds of knowledge: knowledge of the machine, which is physical science; and knowledge of the self, which is not physical science but nevertheless genuine knowledge. He finds this knowledge in literature; but that is only one area of human self-expression in which data about knowledge of the self are to be found. We cannot accept that any area of genuine knowledge can be left outside the boundaries of science. In fact, we believe that the systematic study of the self, the subjective personal experience of human beings, must now be recognized as an enlargement of the boundaries of science. Phillips' "psychological psychology, the study of mankind as subjects," covers a larger field of experience than psychoanalysis. It includes the investigation of intelligence, abilities, individual differences of all kinds, the learning processes in skill acquirement, habit formation, and much more. But his point of view is entirely compatible with that of psychoanalysis, which, because of its basically clinical purpose (the treatment of the emotionally disturbed and ill), has to concentrate on the emotional and motivational dynamics of the personal self in personal relationships. I am here asserting that psychoanalytic therapy provides an even deeper source of data of knowledge of the self than Bronowski's literature, for here we are in firsthand contact with suffering persons who will only allow their worst sufferings to be uncovered with someone in whom they have a hope of finding genuine help. Great literature is saturated with psychopathology. Indeed many great writers and artists were profoundly disturbed and even eventually insane. But they possessed a genius for self-expression, and their tortured experiences tumbled out as they described the sufferings of their fictional heroes and heroines. In psychoanalytic therapy we can share with the patient, at firsthand, the systematic study of the deepest strata of human suffering, with a view of discovering how it can be relieved by a regrowing of the self in a therapeutic relationship. This is psychodynamic science, the complementary other half of the total field of science, which cannot remain within the narrow limits prescribed by the earliest pseudo-philosophy of scientific materialism.

Professor Sir Cyril Burt, one of Britain's most eminent psychologists, stated that, whereas in 1950 most scientists would have dismissed the idea that mind and consciousness should be taken seriously as a phenomenon in its own right, now the issue is reopened. He writes: "In *Brain and Mind* (Smythies. 1965) three of the four neurologists came out in strong support of an uncompromising dualism . . . an unexpected revival of interest in what Schrödinger called 'the most important problem science has yet to face.' " [5] The brain is being regarded as a two-way transmitter and detector, not a generator of consciousness. He cites Penfield as "remaining a dualist rather than an epiphenominalist. It is (Penfield) agrees 'hard to conceive that our being should consist of two separate elements—body and mind: but it is equally incomprehensible that there should be only one element presenting itself as two.' " [6] Burt cites Lord Adrian as saying: "For many of us still one thing seems to lie outside the tidy and familiar (materialist) framework—the 'I' who does the perceiving, the thinking, the acting," [7] and Professor Mace as writing: "Freud seems to have been almost the first to take *mental* determinism seriously as a basic explanation in psychology." [8] Burt himself concludes:

A man's conscious life forms just one continuous event . . . This unity and continuity strongly suggest that the constituent events are related to some permanent and central entity, an entity of a special non-material kind, in short a personal self, who owns these events, and refers to them as *my* conscious experiences or states, and describes himself by the proper name of "I".[9]

Thus the climate of physical science thinking is now calling for a truly mental and personalistic psychology. To Burt's "conscious mind" we have but to add the "unconscious" and we have the field of psychoanalytic investigation.

This ferment of ideas in the wider scientific and cultural climate was unknown in Freud's day. Had it existed then, he would have been able to free himself far more completely from the rigidities of what was held to be true science at that time. Meanwhile, psychoanalysis has developed under the internal pressures of its own clinical experiences and is now in a position to take advantage of the changes that have been going on around it. The claim must be firmly staked for the creation of a psychodynamic science, which could have friendly and cooperative relationships with a general psychology that has outgrown the narrow vision of the behaviorist experimental psychology of recent years. The undisputed starting point of the modern psychodynamic study of the human personality in its emotional, motivational, and human relations living is the work of Freud from 1890 to 1938. Its subsequent development has been due to the interaction of inquiring minds on a worldwide scale, many of them now outside the more narrowly organized psychoanalytic movement. It has spread even into the trained social and educational work of the "helping professions." In a book of this size it is impossible to mention the contributions of many of the most important workers in this field. I have omitted Jung, even though Freudians and Jungians have made some attempts to define their common ground. Jung's intuitive genius leaped ahead to insights, many of which are now being reached by the steady, plodding research of the analysts. I would like to have dealt more fully with the work of Harry Stack Sullivan. It is known that Melanie Klein would have welcomed the opportunity to discuss both men with him. Much might have come of this, for some of his basic concepts, as I have indicated, were of the greatest importance for developing thought in this area.

Otherwise, I have confined myself to psychoanalytic thinkers, for the psychoanalytic movement must be acknowledged as the most important single driving force in this field of investigation. The few names included in the chapter headings will not, I think, be questioned as representing preeminently the particular lines of development I have sought to trace. There is not, however, now or ever, any possibility of treating the study of the many faceted phenomena of our human nature as the monopolistic preserve of any one profession or school of thought. The organic, behavioral, and psychodynamic sciences must learn to recognize each other's contributions and their own limitations, and learn to cooperate. Within the narrower ambit of the psychodynamic field, any tendency to preserve exclusive schools of theory as closed in-groups must spell the death of open-minded scientific inquiry and gravely hinder progress. What I have sought to do here is to trace the growth of psychoanalysis from its nineteenth-century beginnings as a physically based psychophysiology and psychobiology, to a twentieth-century exploration of a new area in an over-all enlarged field of science, psychodynamics. Psychodynamics is defined as the study of the motivated and meaningful life of human beings, as persons shaped in the media of personal relationships which constitute their lives and determine to so large an extent how their innate gifts and possibilities will develop and how, to use Donald Winnicott's terms, the "maturational processes" develop in the "facilitating" or so often "unfacilitating environment" of the other important human beings.

NOTES

1. Martin James, "Psychoanalysis and Childhood, 1967," *The Psychoanalytic Approach*, ed. J. Sutherland (1968).
2. Max Hammerton, "Freud: The Status of an Illusion," *The Listener* (August 29, 1968).
3. R. Phillips, "Psychological Psychology: A New Science?" *The Bulletin of the British Psychological Society* (April, 1968): pp. 83–87.
4. *Ibid.*

5. Cyril Burt, "Brain and Consciousness," *The Bulletin of the British Psychological Society* (1968): pp. 29–36.

6. *Ibid.*

7. *Ibid.*

8. *Ibid.*

9. Cyril Burt, "The Structure of the Mind," *British Journal of Statistical Psychology*, 14 (1961): pp. 145–170.

Chapter 2

THE
STARTING POINT
OF PSYCHODYNAMIC
INQUIRY

FREUD

═══

Since, under the stimulus of day-to-day clincial work in which patients are constantly presenting fresh and unexpected sidelights on familiar problems, it is impossible for one's theoretical position to remain static, I welcome this opportunity of reviewing and bringing up to date the theoretical standpoint that I presented in 1961 in *Personality Structure and Human Interaction* [1] and further developed over the intervening years, in the manuscript prepared for *Schizoid Problems, Object-Relations and the Self*.[2] Since that manuscript was completed early in 1967, I realized that already, in some respects, further clarifications of basic ideas had taken place, and that I would benefit by a further attempt at a condensed statement of the essentials of present-day psychodynamic theory as I see it.

I shall, therefore, at the outset, outline my over-all plan. Perhaps the most important thing I wish to emphasize is that I shall present the "Object-Relations Theory," not as a British School of Psychoanalysis but as a far more fundamental phenomenon. It is true that in *The American Handbook of Psychiatry*, I had the opportunity to present the views of W. R. D. Fairbairn under that heading, and in the broad context of that most comprehensive standard work, there was justification for so doing.[3] Nevertheless, I wish now to place Fairbairn in *his* true context, as part of a long-standing and ongoing movement of thought in the psychodynamic exploration of human nature. I shall thus describe object-relations theory as the struggle for predominance of one of the two different types of thinking mixed and confused together in psychoanalysis from its earliest beginnings in the work of Freud. Object-relations theory, or to use the American version, "Interpersonal-Relations Theory," is the emancipation of Freud's psychodynamic personal thinking from its bondage to his natural-science, impersonal, intellectual heritage. We must, therefore, look again at the clash of neurophysiology, psychobiology, and psychodynamics in the arena of Freud's restlessly original and exploratory mind. There has never been a stage of psychoanalytic theorizing when both lines of thought have not been visible, but gradually research into the ego and personal relationships has more and more occupied the center of the stage.

While Hartmann has elaborately modernized classic psychobiology, others both in Britain and America have been developing the personal, psychodynamic implications of Freud's work. While the work of Karen Horney, Erich Fromm, Clara Thompson, and others revealed the onesidedness of Freud's too exclusively biological theory, and forced social factors to be taken more specifically into account, Harry Stack Sullivan's clear rejection of instinct as an adequate concept for human psychology, and his adoption of interpersonal relations experience as his basic concept, I believe as early as 1925, was the first absolute breakthrough of object-relations theory. It must have seemed far more disconcerting to psychoanalysts in general at that time, than it could do now, and the limitations of Sullivan's theory are today more clear. Nevertheless, it was a challenging and important advance outside of the official psychoanalytic movement.

In Chapter 3 I shall seek to show how the work of Melanie Klein became, in a subtle way (closely related to depth psychology), the unwitting originator of a similar major reorientation in the direction of object-relations theory from inside the psychoanalytic movement. From that time on, this stream of thought broadened irresistibly. In distinction to the system-ego of Freud and Hartmann, a person-ego theory grew steadily in the work of W. R. D. Fairbairn and Erik Erikson, and is now coming to fruition in the work of Donald Winnicott and others in the child therapy field. The person-ego theory shows how the very beginnings of ego growth as the core of selfhood in the psyche as a whole person is entirely bound up with the first and fundamental object-relationship, that of the mother and her baby. This, then, is the ground I shall try to cover, and at the outset I must make three qualifying remarks.

1. As already stated, I do not regard object-relations theory as a new school of psychoanalysis. In thinking about human nature, it is too easy to have an emotional investment in our theory. In this field, the formation of rival schools, in-groups, too self-contained theories, is surely a betraying sign of anxiety. There is something wrong with us if our theoretical ideas remain stagnant and impervious to change for too long. Theory is simply the best we can do to date to conceptualize the experiences our patients present to us. Winnicott once wrote that it is impossible for an analyst to be original, for what he writes today, he learned (from a patient) yesterday. In fact, we have to beware of imposing our fixed ideas on our

patients. I suppose every analyst of any amount of experience, can remember how, in the early days, he would at times interpret according to the book and fail to get any response from the patient. We could not do without theoretical guidelines, most of all in the days of inexperience, but it is not as easy as some critics think to impose on the patient ideas that don't fit or are irrelevant at that particular moment. The ideal time for interpretation has always been stated to be the moment when the patient is almost seeing something for himself and needs help to overcome some last bit of resistance. As analytical experience increases, the analyst is more likely to have the experience of a patient saying, "It is strange you should say that: I did think something like that only this morning." But there is never a stage at which patients do not make some remarks that throw subtle new light on old problems. If we are receptive, this keeps our theory moving and alive. Before I came to psychoanalysis in practice, a rigorous training in philosophy made me skeptical about all theories. Clearly human thought never reaches finality. I came to the conclusion that particularly theories about human nature always represent a modicum of fact described within the limits of the cultural outlook of some one restricted period of social history. It is easy to show how this was true of Freud, or of Victorian science as represented by Thomas H. Huxley, or of the new learning theory and behavior therapy as represented in Britain by Hans Eysenck. At least Huxley had the insight to qualify his views about scientific materialism and epiphenominalism, or the view that mind is only like the steam whistle on a train and has no real influence, by the significantly wistful comment "Perhaps I am color-blind" about these things.

In a review of "Depth Psychology: A Critical History," by Dieter Wyss, Leon Salzman says, "Two histories of psychoanalysis are combined in this volume." One of them is that of the vicissitudes of "a theory of behavior in the then prevailing model of energy mechanics and oversimplified concepts of causality. . . . The most rigid psychoanalytic theorists, insisting on the maintenance of all of Freud's original speculations, in the long run destroy their possibilities." The other history is that of the efforts to "move personality theory closer to a valid statement about man and his psychology. . . . The physical models which have been offered to date do not adequately encompass man, who functions through a system of values as well as physiochemical changes." [4] Salzman adds two important comments to this.

Psychoanalysis is a science, not a religion or a system of beliefs which required dedicated loyalty and ritualistic worship. The institutionalization of psychoanalytic training and the organization of associations designed to maintain the purity of theory and the status of its practitioners have been most damaging to the prospects of an ultimate personality theory based upon psychodynamic principles. It is certain that the essential contributions of Freud which relate to the dynamic concept of personality development, the influence of early experiencing the role out-of-awareness factors in human behaviour, and the technique for exploring introspective and subjective experiencing will remain.[5]

It is in exactly Salzman's spirit that I shall seek to disentangle the two coexisting strands in Freud's thought. Freud himself showed a mind that was forever on the move, one of the things we have most cause to be grateful to him for. He had the courage to change his own theories again and again. Joan Riviere once wrote "In 1924, when I was struggling with obscurities in 'The Ego and the Id' for translation, and pestered Freud to give me clearer expression of his meaning, he answered me, exasperated, 'The book will be obsolete in thirty years.' " [6] Freud gave us a starting point—theories that contain elements of permanent value—and also a tremendous example of not becoming bogged down just there, but rather of going on gathering new experiences and experimenting with new hypotheses.

2. For this reason also, the term "object-relations theory"

should not be limited to the work of Fairbairn. He would have been horrified at the idea of founding a new school of psychoanalysis. He contributed seminal ideas to the common stock of understanding. When Parkinson's disease and cerebral thrombosis claimed him as their victim, they prevented him from completing his work. He had intended to write and had gathered material for a full-scale study of hysteria. He had outlined to me some ideas he was developing on the nature of psychoanalysis as science. I regretted not having made notes of that conversation, as I was not able to get him to go over that ground again. When he read the first draft of my paper on ego-weakness soon afterward, he said, "I'm glad you've written this. If I could write now, this is what I would be writing about." It was sad to see this man who knew that he had more to give, while increasing weakness robbed him of the power to express it. I owe much to the inspiration of his thought and have done something to develop it, but I feel bound to honor the spirit of this man and say that I am not a "Fairbairnian" and that there is no such thing. He did not think in such terms. What there is is not a school of thought but a steadily developing concentration on "the personal ego in object-relations." Fairbairn, deriving stimulus from Melanie Klein, made an outstanding contribution to this area, although he did not provide a dogma but a stimulus to research.

The term "object-relations theory" should not therefore be limited to Fairbairn's work. In the 1940s and early 1950s he did call his work object-relationships theory, implying not a new theory, but a deliberate emphasis on the personal side of Freud's theory of parent-child (Oedipal) relations. Tavistock clinic sympathizers suggested the shorter form "object-relations theory." Ian Suttie, in his "Origins of Love and Hate," an early Tavistock man, was in a sense a forerunner of Fairbairn, who once said to me, "Suttie really had something important to say." The truth, however, is that important ideas grow in particular subtle atmospheres of thought. Fairbairn could not have written as he did at the end of the last century nor in the first two decades of this one. In those days Freud was struggling to break out of the rigid enclosure of natural science without ceasing to be scientific, so as to found psychoanalysis, or as I would prefer to call it in this context, psychodynamic science. The resulting subtle changes in the climate of thought that were begun by Freud liberated original minds to develop further changes, Harry Stack Sullivan, Melanie Klein, and Ronald Fairbairn being among them. Only in historical perspective can we think realistically about these matters; certainly not in terms of defending or attacking any schools of thought.

Object-relations theory, or rather object-relational thinking, is a broad stream of thought today. Its roots may be found in the work of Freud on the Oedipus complex and the phenomena of transference and resistance in treatment. It expanded tremendously in the work of Melanie Klein on internal objects, became explicitly conscious of itself in American psychosociology and in Fairbairn's correlations of internal-object-splittings and ego-splittings, has been clinically developed in Erikson's ego-identity studies, and in the most radical way deepened by Winnicott's work on ego-origins in the earliest mother-infant relationships. These outstanding names represent a developing movement in which large numbers of people, both inside and outside the psychoanalytic organization, have taken part. As one who is not a member of any psychoanalytical society, though working by the psychoanalytic method and trained in it by Fairbairn and Winnicott, I feel it is proper to say that, with one or two exceptions, by far the major debt owed by all of us is to the psychoanalytic movement that sustains an organized mass of research. Yet today, even the psychoanalytic movement is not ideologically homogeneous, and not all of it contributes to object-relations theory. In fact, object-relational thinking is now not an organization but a broad movement of thought that belongs to this age in a special manner, as a counterbalancing movement to the enormous growth of physical science. A main spur to its development is the necessity to provide a counterpoise to diametrically opposed theories that are nondynamic, nonobject-relational, and nonpersonal and that seek to impose natural science thought-forms on the study of the intimate and personal life of man; generally by taking note only of symptoms and ignoring the meaning and values of subjective experience. As I sought to show in Chapter 1, the existence of two different psychologies, dynamic and nondynamic, does not necessarily imply that they must be opposed. All such opposition is essentially unscientific. But when opposition does occur (and my impression is that hitherto psychoanalysts have been more ready to accept that there is a place for behavior therapy than the behaviorists have been ready to recognize that there is a place for psychoanalysis), then it is symptomatic of the cultural predicament of our time, and represents life as persons having to fight for survival in an age dominated by purely objective, mechanistic science and technology. Psychodynamic thinkers are then obliged to carry the fight into the camp of traditional science and show its incapacity for dealing with psychic reality.

3. My last qualifying remark, which I feel must be made in view of the wide sweep of psychoanalytic territory surveyed, is that I cannot claim to be in any sense a psychoanalytic polymath, or to have read everything that is important in this field. The literature is now so extensive that it would take a psychoanalytic historian, devoted solely to the scholarly study of the entire movement, to cope with it. But there is another reason. To devote too much time to scholarship would be to have too little time to treat patients, which is the important thing, and as a result would stifle one's own independent thinking. We must find guiding ideas from books and from one another, but it is from patients that we learn the facts about human nature at firsthand, taking into account our

own personal analysis. I have chosen rather to study a few writers who seemed to me to stand out as truly creative, such as Sullivan, Melanie Klein, Fairbairn, Erikson, Hartmann, and Winnicott. There are papers by Karl Abraham, Sandor Ferenczi, and Ernest Jones that no one can afford not to read. I owe a debt to Marjorie Brierley not only for her writings and her stimulus in personal discussion but also for her bringing into the psychoanalytic arena the concept of personology, an ugly word but an indispensable idea. Both the lectures of J. C. Flügel, in my undergraduate days, and his scholarly writings have been invaluable. There are others I would fain have had time to read thoroughly, but have only been able to dip into their work, along with their contributions to *The International Journal* that arrested my attention. I take this opportunity of acknowledging my indebtedness to articles in *The International Journal* by Maxwell Gitelson, Leo Rangell, Robert Holt, and especially Bernard Apfelbaum for enabling me to see the work of Heinz Hartmann and the ego-psychology movement he stimulated, through various and differing American eyes. But it seems to me that, once grounded in the fundamentals of theory, the important thing is to be constantly testing ideas by the evidence that patients bring. To care for people is more important than to care for ideas, which can be good servants but bad masters, and my interests have always been primarily in clinical work rather than in theory as such. The survey of theory that follows no doubt omits much that is important but it is close to, and primarily reflects, what I am able to see actually going on in disturbed human beings seeking help.

Whatever one has or has not read, there is one must. We all *must* begin with Freud, because he is the starting point for Freudians, neo-Freudians, and even for non-Freudians and anti-Freudians alike; no one can ignore or bypass Freud. In the early days Jung, Adler, and Rank were all profoundly affected by him. Melanie Klein and Fairbairn, Hartmann and

Erikson all regarded themselves as both developing and, also in various ways, going beyond Freud. For the moment it is enough to say that Hartmann developed Freud's system-ego theory in new directions, while the object-relational views so greatly stimulated by Klein's work have led rather to the conceptualization of a person-ego theory. It is a not insignificant historical accident that Hartmann came to America while Melanie Klein came to Britain, for in spite of the apparent orthodoxy of her instinct theory, it was Melanie Klein's work that so greatly stimulated object-relational thinking in Britain. As I have explained, it is my purpose to show that this can mislead us, and that object-relational thinking must be studied as a movement of thought inherent in psychoanalysis from its inception. If it is not as prominent in Hartmann as it is in the work of some others in America, it is still there, and a stimulating cross-fertilization of ideas in psychodynamics is taking place today between those studying these matters on both sides of the Atlantic.

Freud's ideas fall into two main groups, (1) the id-plus-ego-control apparatus, and (2) the Oedipus complex of family object-relationship situations with their reappearance in treatment as transference and resistance. The first group of ideas tends to picture the psyche as a mechanism, an impersonal arrangement for securing detensioning, a homeostatic organization. The second group tends toward a personal psychology of the influence people have on each other's lives, particularly parents on children. This second group of ideas led Freud beyond the study of sex, with its obvious biological basis and function, to aggression, with its obvious social concomitants of guilt and depression, and so to the concept of the superego, an aspect of psychic life not traceable to biology but based on identification with parents. The superego enshrines the fact of personal object-relations, since Freud pointed out that the overcoming of the Oedipus complex is effected by identification taking the place of Oedipal relations with parents. It is thus highly significant that in Hartmann's work the superego declines in importance with all of its object-relational connotations and falls into the background behind the autonomous system-ego and its apparatuses. In the work of Melanie Klein, the superego is actually the starting point of all of her new developments. Hartmann has developed to the full the more impersonal aspect of Freud's theory, while Melanie Klein developed the object-relational aspect. R. and K. Eissler, in their contribution to the Hartmann *Festschrift*, show him to be a mind in the true classical mold, not only a methodical and most painstaking thinker but also a man of mature and wide scholarship on the basis of a very thorough scientific education. He was ideally suited to the task of developing and completing the more impersonal ego-apparatus ideas of Freud, tracing them through all of their many changes, as he does for example with Freud's concept of the ego in Chapter 14 of *Essays on Ego Psychology*. In this he carried the work of Freud to its utmost limits of elaboration, drawing out implications that Freud himself had no time or opportunity to explore. But Hartmann remains in a fundamental way orthodox from the point of view of the classical psychoanalytical tradition, in spite of his autonomous ego concept. It is not simply that he retained the concept of the Id, for in varying degrees Melanie Klein, Erickson, and even Winnicott continue to use that term. It is rather that Hartmann's theory never really comes to life as a dynamic psychology of whole and unique persons. Rather he seeks to make contacts with general psychology, which today tends markedly to be nondynamic and nonpersonal. Just as the behavior therapist's human being is simply a repertoire of behavior patterns, a personality-pattern but not a real person or self, so in Hartmann the ego is a repertoire of apparatuses and automatisms for internal control and for external adaptation to outer reality but not a personal self. The person is taken for granted, and all the emphasis is on the system-ego, true to the id-plus-ego-control apparatus aspect of Freud's theory. It is a structural theory, not a personal theory.

We shall do well at this point to remind ourselves of just how impersonal that side of Freud's thought could be, by turning to his *Beyond the Pleasure Principle*. Freud, being the pioneer of an entirely new approach to the study of man, could not have foreseen how deeply he would be involved in a conflict of loyalties between the traditional natural science in which he was raised, which was shaped for the objective study of material phenomena, and the new psychodynamic science, which he was destined to create. The two parts of his theory reflect this, the impersonal apparatus for the control of id-drives (the hydraulic model as it has been called) on the one hand, and the object-relational life of meaningful and motivated relations between persons, beginning with parents and children on the other hand. The impersonal aspect of Freud's theory was developed in the interests of being scientific, and we know that Freud's first attempt at large-scale theory construction was purely neurophysiological, as in *Project for a Scientific Psychology* or *Psychology for Neurologists* in 1895. When he found that its concepts did not explain truly psychological phenomena, Freud had the courage to drop the scheme and move on to experiment with other biological ideas. The new learning theorists of today may believe that they have succeeded where Freud failed, but, in fact, they occupy in all essentials that same position that he rejected as inadequate. I am not saying that their studies of conditioning, habit-forming, and reconditioning are invalid. That would not be true, and I accept the fact that their type of study ought to be carried on. But I hold Freud to be right when he decided that it is not psychology, and it was a psychology that he was really in search of.

In the second great phase of his theory-making, Freud turned to the concept of instincts, which looked to be sufficiently psychological. Although he did once write, "Instincts are our mythology," Freud never really abandoned his psychobiology. Nevertheless, from about 1915 to 1920 onward, the strong wine of Freud's relentless quest began once more to burst the bottles of old theory. It drove him on to ego-analysis, but because this remained tied to his psychobiology, we must look more closely into it. It was still basically far more a natural science type of theorizing than a truly personal one. Freud was trying to ride two horses at once, that of mechanistic theory with his economic and topographical points of view, and that of personal theory in his dynamic point of view worked out on the basis of psychogenetic processes in the medium of family relationships. Although even Freud's dynamic drives oscillated between being biochemical and psychological energies, the concept of psychic energy is a difficult one to work with because the concept of energy belongs to physical science.

In *Beyond the Pleasure Principle*, Freud speaks of his views as speculative assumptions, but somehow they come to be treated as facts.

The course taken by mental events is automatically regulated by the pleasure principle. . . . The course of those events is invariably set in motion by an unpleasurable tension, and . . . it takes a direction such that its final outcome coincides with a lowering of that tension—that is with an avoidance of unpleasure or a production of pleasure.[7]

Note the term "automatically," which is mechanistic, not psychologically meaningful. The mental or what should be the psychologically significant terms, "pleasure and unpleasure," turn out to be not really relevant, for Freud goes on to say:

We have decided to relate pleasure and unpleasure to the quantity of excitation that is present in the mind . . . and to relate them in such a manner that unpleasure corresponds to an *increase* in the quantity of excitation, and pleasure to a *diminution*.[8]

It is clear that these views, to use Freud's words, come from "all that we have been taught by psychophysiology."

The facts which have caused us to believe in the dominance of the pleasure principle in mental life, also find expression in the hypothesis that the mental apparatus endeavours to keep the quantity of mental excitation in it as low as possible or at least to keep it constant. This latter hypothesis is only another way of stating the pleasure principle. . . . The pleasure principle flows. from the constancy principle.[9]

This constancy principle was defined by Breuer and Freud in their *Studies in Hysteria,* as the "tendency to maintain intra-cerebral excitation at a constant level." That there is a subtle confusion of two different types of thought here, is shown in Freud's expression "the mental apparatus endeavours." If there is "endeavour," that is, purposive striving, then we are on psychological ground and are not dealing with an apparatus but with a motivated psychic self. If, however, there is an apparatus, that is a mechanistic concept and the use of the term "endeavor" is out of place.

This pleasure or constancy principle, which became known to physiologists later as "homeostasis," valuable as it is for the functioning of the organism, becomes misleading when used to explain our lives as persons. A psychic self devoted to keeping the quantity of excitation at as low a level as possible and constant, that is, unvarying, would in our everyday lives be a recipe for boredom. It is too like the mother who is always saying "Now then, don't get too excited. If you laugh like that, you'll be crying in a minute." Victorian young ladies, brought up on the "constancy principle," or as it was then termed the "modesty principle," found a blind escape into what were called "the vapours." Increased excitation, far from being always experienced as unpleasure, is more usually experienced as relief from dullness, when our personal experience rather than just physiology is considered. When people are incapable of genuine enjoyment, they usually fly to excitation as a substitute for it. This physiological quantity theory in fact reduced any psychological consciousness of experiences to the level of a mere accompaniment of bodily processes, exactly what Huxley meant when he called "mind" an epiphenomenon. This is not psychology at all, but brain physiology. When it strays out of its proper place, it becomes brain-philosophy, or scientific materialism. We do not encounter much writing of this kind in psychoanalysis today, though Holt seems to want to recall us to it, and psychologists are still pursuing inquiries on that level. It is a valid inquiry as long as it does not claim to be more than it is, that is, psychophysiology, a study of the physical basis of mental or psychic life. It is not psychology, a study of mental or psychic life in its own right. We should not forget how really nonpsychological and impersonal was *one side* of Freud's basic theorizing, representing all that he was being driven to transcend. But the greatness of Freud was just that his emotional intuition and his intellectual urge to exploration could not be bound by his professional scientific education.

We may turn with relief from this obstructive loyalty to physical science in a field where it fails to explain what we want to understand, and then come upon the object-relations side of Freud's thought. This was the source of all that was most creative in his work. Ernest Jones thought that the first half of Freud's theorizing represented a closed and completed whole, and that Freud made a completely new start when he turned to structural theory and ego analysis. I think it is more truthful to say that the change represents the partially successful struggle of the object-relational element in Freud's insight to break through the straightjacket of traditional scientific physical thought-forms. Object-relational thinking is the emancipation of the core of psychodynamic insight. This was the inner driving-force in psychoanalytic thinking from the earliest moment when Freud became dissatisfied with the understanding of neurosis implied in the hydropathic and other empirical and useless treatments of his day, and began to probe and question with one of the most fearless minds ever brought to bear on human problems. It is true that his object-relational insight had to become disentangled from his inherited theory of instinct-physiology. This really began, although it was not realized for a long time, when Freud moved beyond the sex instinct to add a second major instinct of aggression; for whatever aggression is, it is certainly not an instinct in the same sense as sex. This vague and variably defined term "instinct" is akin to the term "faculty." As early as 1931 Fairbairn wrote:

The general tendency of modern science is to throw suspicion upon entities: and it was under the influence of that tendency that the old "faculty-psychology" perished. *Perhaps the arrangement of mental phenomena into functioning structure groups is the most that can be attempted by psychological science.* [Present writer's italics]. At any rate it would appear contrary to the spirit of modern science to confer the status of entity upon "instincts," and in the light of modern knowledge an instinct seems best regarded as a characteristic dynamic pattern of behaviour.[10]

I prefer, with Fairbairn and Sullivan to abandon the use of the term "instinct" (though Fairbairn would use the adjective "instinctive," but not the noun "instinct," to safeguard against reification and entity-making). Perhaps today he would have felt that the term "pattern of behavior" was too impersonal and static in its behavioristic implications, even when prefixed by the adjective "dynamic." He later gave up the use of the term "libido" for the same reason and spoke always of the libidinal ego. He held that so-called instincts are not entities, and certainly "not forces invading the ego from outside itself, giving it a kick in the pants," but dynamic reactions of a "person-ego," sexually or aggressively, in and to an object-relational situation. Even so, there is a fundamental difference between sexual and aggressive ego-reactions to objects. With sex, the quality of mental experience and the ensuing behavior arise initially from a physical, biochemical state of the organism. With aggression, it is the other way round. The biochemical state accompanying aggressive reactions results from a mental emotional experience. To put this in a wider context, sex belongs to the phenomena we group together as "appetites," with hunger, thirst, excretion, breathing (need for air), and probably sleep and the need for physical exercise. The appetites are all concerned primarily with the survival and reproduction of the bodily organism and are not concerned primarily with the needs of the personal psyche. The appetites *can* all be endowed with personal-relationship significance, and this is most easily done with sex, hunger, thirst, and exercise. Obsessional mothers manage to endow excretion with a great deal of unnecessary guilt-burdened personal-relations meaning. The same may happen to breathing when a smothering mother drives her daughter into asthma, as happened to one of my patients. This patient was also held to be allergic to feather cushions, but it turned out that it was only her mother's cushions that upset her. Sleep acquires a profound personal-relations significance when the ability to go to sleep in the presence of another person expresses a feeling of security in relation to that person. Thus toward the end of a successful analysis it can be a good sign if the patient can relax and go to sleep in a session. On one such occasion the patient said "Something has healed in me deep down." On the other hand, a male patient said that the only time he had ever been to bed with a woman—he did not mind trying it, to see what it was like—he was terrified to go to sleep. Later he broke his only engagement when he found that his fiancée took it for granted that they would sleep in a double bed. He had a really dominating mother who had overlaid his personality. Similarly, the need for physical exercise can be endowed with a personal-relations significance, as when it is turned into competitive athletic sports where physical prowess is a tremendous ego-booster in relation to other people. There is no need to stress the tremendous extent to which eating and drinking are endowed with a personal-relations significance as being symbolic of friendship and sharing. Thus the bodily appetites or needs can be and practically always are endowed with highly personal values as forms of relating to other people, but they can in fact be satisfied simply as bodily needs with no further meaning. The more excretory functions are disentangled from personal relationships and freed to function simply as a private biological elimination of waste matter, accompanied by a mild, private sensuous pleasure, the healthier it is. It is possible to eat and drink alone for no other reason than that one is hungry or thirsty, and it is optional to make eating and drinking a social matter.

Of all the appetites, sex is the only one that cannot be wholly divorced from object-relations, which is why it is so much caught up and involved in psychoneuroses; though even then it is possible for sexual relations to be more physical than personal. Those who cannot make genuinely personal relations often fall back on bodily sexual relations as a substitute, only to find that sex does not fill the aching mental void. One male patient of a very schizoid aloof type said that he had no real sex life, but only what he called "an intermittent biological urge which has nothing to do with me," which he simply satisfied with a prostitute. Another male patient who superficially was the very opposite of this, having lived quite promiscuously for a number of years, came for treatment for depression, which was really apathy. He said "I think this sex business is a much over-rated pleasure. I'm bored with it." He seemed really surprised when I suggested that that was bound to be the case, since none of the women he had been with had meant anything to him at all. Neither of these two patients had any real personal relationships. Thus we must regard Freud's sex instinct as basically an appetite, primarily subserving an organic need for reproduction, but, because of its essentially cooperative nature, it is an appetite that is especially capable of being taken up into the life of the person in relation to another person. The brain and the genitals are the two points at which most clearly biological needs for organs that facilitate survival and psychological needs for effecting relationships as persons meet together, but there is no more reason for calling sex an instinct than there would be for calling perceiving and thinking instincts. This particular appetite of sex, however, though it is basically a matter of physiology, can only function satisfactorily when it *is* satisfied in the service of a mature and responsible person in genuine personal relationship. Otherwise sex ends up as a source of disillusionment.

For the moment I am most interested in making the point that in sex we start with a biochemical state of the body, an organic appetite, which is then either taken up into or else excluded from the life of personal relationship. In sharp contrast, aggression is not primarily a dynamic organic pattern of behavior; it is rather a dynamic personal pattern of behavior, taking its origin in an emotional reaction of anger, itself a result of fear of some danger, both of which are emotional experiences that stimulate biochemical changes in the body. Aggression is a personal meaningful reaction to bad-object relations, to a threat to the ego, aroused initially by fear. If there is nothing to fear, there is nothing to fight. Aggression is a defensive anger in a situation in which the menace is not too great for us to cope with. Otherwise aggression changes into frustrated rage, hate, fear, and flight. The accompanying biochemical changes are the result, not the cause, of the mental state. Sex is primarily biological and then becomes personal, aggression is primarily personal and then becomes biological. Thus, another important contrast between sex and aggression is that the appetites have a regular organic periodicity. Aggression has no regular periodicity, but is related simply to the personal object-relations situation. To sum up, the clear difference between sex and aggression, showing that they cannot both be regarded as instincts in Freud's sense, may be put thus: sex, as a bodily appetite, is concerned primarily with bodily aims, however much it can be and is taken up into the service of personal aims, while aggression, as a defensive reaction to a threat to the ego, is concerned primarily with personal aims, however much it may be secondarily used in the service of organic self-preservation as the basis of the personal life. Sex serves the organism first and the personal self second, while aggression reverses this and serves the personal self first and the organism second. It is because of this that when Freud's interest moved beyond sex to aggression, (and beyond hysteria to guilt, obsessional neurosis and depression), the personal, object-relational side of his thinking, always clearly present in the Oedipal theory, came to the forefront, and impersonal psychophysiology and psychobiology began to fall into the background without this being explicitly recognized. His third phase of thinking concentrated on ego-analysis, group psychology, the superego, and all object-relational phenomena. He now ceased to regard anxiety as dammed up sexual libido converted into tension, and saw it realistically as an ego-reaction to danger, to bad-objects.

The original instinct theory remained, however, to slow down progress, still being regarded as the foundation of ego-psychology. Yet the difference between sex and aggression was now tacitly admitted in Freud's structural theory in which sex-drives were regarded as emerging from the hypothetical id to plague the ego, but aggression was taken up into the superego to strengthen ego-control in view of social demands. There is a striking difference here between Freud and Plato, and it is Plato who is the more consistent thinker. In distinguishing between sex and aggression, Plato gives aggression the more personal role as the admired courageous soldier defending the citadel of reason in the ego, against the dangerous many-headed beast of the lusts and passions of the flesh. Freud, believing it essential to maintain the view that aggression is an instinct, a so-called id-drive, could only do this by degrading it into innate destructiveness, and inventing one of his most unfortunate concepts, that of the death instinct, which Fenichel, Jones, and almost all analysts except Kleinians rejected. Hartmann tried to save this situation by drawing a distinction between (1) aggression as a primary drive on the same level as sexuality, and (2) Freud's speculation about Eros and Thanatos, which he holds to be biological mysticism, a biological hypothesis as distinct from the first, which he regards as a clinical hypothesis.[11] Within the terms of Freud's own theorizing, that distinction is correct (a fact that we shall see is important in interpreting Melanie Klein's work), but it does not help us with our present problem, not only because sex and Eros, aggression and Thanatos came to be treated as identical by those analysts who accepted the death instinct but also because clinically, aggression simply is not "a primary drive on the same level as sexuality"; it is a personal defensive reaction against a threat to the ego. I believe that Freud's failure to differentiate properly between sex and aggression is the main reason why psychoanalytic theory has taken so long to disentangle biology and psychodynamics; and to realize that its real business is to create a consistently psychodynamic ego-theory of man as a whole person, developing our true nature in the medium of those personal object-relations that alone give meaning to our lives. The most striking clinical proof of this is the full-scale schizoid person for whom object-loss involves ego-loss, and whose only "affect" if it can be called such is that feeling of "futility" that Fairbairn pinpointed as characteristic of this state. When the ego is lost, the so-called id-drives cease to drive, and this leads to schizoid suicide because there is no longer any point in going on living.

The practical consequences of Freud's instinct theory are

serious for psychotherapy. The analyst can blame failure on the supposedly too great constitutional strength of the patient's sex or more likely aggression. While we certainly cannot "cure" everyone, I believe that such failures are more likely to result from the thearpist's failure to give a relationship in which the patient feels secure enough to go beyond his aggression and bring his isolation to the therapist. I have never yet met any patient whose overintense sexuality and/or agression could not be understood in object-relational terms, as resulting from too great and too early deprivations of mothering and general frustration of healthy development in his childhood. Pathological sex and aggression can then be seen as actually the persistence of the infant's struggle to become a viable ego, a personal self, by means of both good and bad object-relating. This implies a person-ego theory as distinct from Hartmann's system-ego theory. His structural psychology is of a particular kind, which treats psychic structures as almost being entities in themselves. Since Hartmann does not stress the superego, we are almost left with a dualistic theory of human nature, an id and an ego, id-drives and an ego over against them that is partly a control apparatus, and partly over and above that an autonomous ego developing in a conflict-free area of the psyche, its own techniques of *adaptation* to outer reality. Edward Glover in a work written in 1961 regarded this as static and mechanistic.

Hartmann's theory is really determined by the fact that he accepted, as its basis, Freud's id-drives as primary energies apart from and outside the ego. Being eminently a logical and consistent thinker, he could then only develop an ego-concept that would be complementary to the impersonal id-drives on the one hand, a system-ego or control apparatus, and on the other hand an organ of adaptation to the environment. In either case this ego is not a person and cannot be a whole self. Bernard Apfelbaum, in a searching critique of this kind of structural theory, saw how difficult it is to keep frank dualism out of it. He wrote of "the isolating tendency inherent in structural thinking. Perhaps any ego psychology assumes or implies a congruent id psychology." [12] It does, unless it is a person-ego theory. The only escape from a dualism of radically opposed structures is to banish the term "id," and reserve "ego" to denote the whole basically unitary psyche with its innate potential for developing into a true self, a whole person, using his psychosomatic energies for self-expression and self-realization in interpersonal relationships. Structural theory can then be used less objectionally in Fairbairn's sense of "the arrangement of mental phenomena into functioning structure groups," to describe "ego-splitting," the internal disharmonies and conflicts and inconsistencies into which the psyche as a whole self is plunged by disturbing and disintegrating bad-object relations in infancy.

This is really the problem of how, realistically, to relate biology and psychodynamics. Hartmann and Fairbairn were both severely logical thinkers though in opposite ways, and in a way Hartmann was as opposed as Fairbairn to a confused mixing of two separate disciplines. Fairbairn accepted the biological inheritance as the basic given, dropped the nonpsychological term "id," and used the term "instinct" only adjectivally to characterize some ego-processes. He was then free to concentrate on the psychology of the ego as a whole person. Hartmann took the opposite line by retaining the id and thus never developed a truly personal psychology, and always sought to discover the basis of his ego-apparatuses in brain-physiology. Had he found them, they would have had nothing to do with the reasons for the motivated actions of persons in real life. Erikson and Winnicott, being less severely logical thinkers, could still use the term "id," though I think inconsistently, but without bothering to subject it to much scrutiny, and left their clinical intuition free to wander in search of the subjective realities of human living. We shall consider the results in Chapters 4 and 5.

41

I regard Sullivan as giving us the correct way to relate biology and psychodynamics, by progressing beyond instinct theory to personal theory. His term, "the biological substrate of personality," is fully adequate to take care of the appetites as organic needs, and the brain and nervous system as the machinery of perception, thinking, control and motility, and of the whole autonomic functioning of the organism, while leaving us free to recognize how they are taken up into the developing psychic self or personal ego. We can thus think of a whole person whose organic appetites and other endowments are owned by and operated within his psychic self or ego. Their mode of operation will be determined by the over-all state of the ego or personal self. An angry, aggressive, hating ego will be sexually sadistic, hungrily devouring (oral sadism), deliberately dirtying and befouling in excretion (anal hate). A frightened ego will be sexually impotent, may be unable to swallow food or develop anorexia nervosa, and will be likely to suffer constipation or retention. A mature, friendly, stable ego will be sexually loving, will find simple pleasure in eating and drinking according to his actual needs and pleasant company, and will leave excretion to function without interference as biological disposal of waste. Clara Thompson wrote of Sullivan's theory of interpersonal relations: "He holds that, given a biological substrate, the human is the product of the interaction with other human beings, that it is out of the personal and social forces acting upon one from the day of birth that the personality emerges." [13] Sullivan himself wrote: "The idea of 'human' instincts in anything like the proper rigid meaning . . . is completely preposterous. All discussion of 'human instincts' is apt to be very misleading and a block to correct thinking, unless the term 'instinct' . . . is so broadened in its meaning that there is no particular sense in using the term at all." [14] One other quotation from Sullivan must be given. "Biological and neurophysiological terms are utterly inadequate for studying everything in life . . . I hope you will not try to build up in your thinking, correlations (that is, 'of "somatic" organization with psychiatrically important phenomena') that are purely imaginary . . . an illusion born out of the failure to recognize that what we know comes to us through our *experiencing* of events." [15] Sullivan's recognition of the *subjectivity of experiencing* as the true concern of psychodynamic studies and his definition of this as interpersonal relations, marks the emergence in the clearest possible way of object-relational thinking disentangled from biology. I remember discussing Sullivan with Fairbairn around the early 1950s, and he stated how close he felt that he and Sullivan were on this basic matter, of moving beyond the impersonal to the personal levels of abstraction, from mechanistic to motivational concepts. It is a great pity that Sullivan and Fairbairn never met. Fairbairn owed far more to Freud than Sullivan did, but they both moved beyond classical psychoanalysis at the same point. Traditional science deals with "events" that have no meaning; they are merely happenings. Psychodynamic science deals with "experiences," meaningful states, and significant relationships. In one single observation, that "the infant empathizes the mother's anxiety," Sullivan anticipated Winnicott's work on the origins of the ego in the mother-infant relationship. We shall look closer at Erikson's views in Chapter 4, but we may say now that Sullivan and Erikson have explored the growth of the individual ego in its ever-widening social milieu, while Melanie Klein, Fairbairn, and Winnicott have delved ever deeper into the internal psychic drama of the growing ego, back to its earliest beginnings. In each case it was the "object-relational" aspect of Freud's thought that was being followed up, not his psychophysiology and psychobiology. What I have tried to show here is that, of the two strands in Freud's thought, the natural science and the *psychodynamic*, the physiological and the *personal*, the mechanistic and the *object-relational*, it was the latter that was struggling to break free and develop in its own right. The story of post-Freudian development is the story of its successful issue. The closer we keep to clinical experience, the more certain is this result. We have to remember that clinical practice does not exist as an arena for the display of psychodynamic theory; rather psychodynamic theory exists to preserve and develop whatever insights we gain in clinical practice.

NOTES

1. Harry Guntrip, *Personality Structure and Human Interaction,* The International Psycho-Analytical Library (London: The Hogarth Press; New York: International Universities Press, 1961).
2. Harry Guntrip, *Schizoid Problems, Object-Relations, and the Self,* The International Psycho-Analytical Library (London: The Hogarth Press; New York: International Universities Press, 1968).
3. Harry Guntrip, "The Object-Relations Theory of W. R. D. Fairbairn," *The American Handbook of Psychiatry,* vol. 3 (New York: Basic Books, 1966), chap. 17.
4. Leon Salzman, *Psychiatry and Social Science Review* 1, no. 12 (1967).
5. *Ibid.*
6. Melanie Klein, et al, *Developments in Psychoanalysis* (London: The Hogarth Press; New York: Hillary House, 1952), p. 1.
7. Sigmund Freud, *Beyond the Pleasure Principle* (London: The Hogarth Press, revised edition, 1959; New York: International Universities Press).
8. *Ibid.,* p. 2.
9. *Ibid.,* p. 4.
10. W. Ronald D. Fairbairn, *An Object-Relations Theory of the Personality* (New York: Basic Books, 1954), p. 218.
11. Heinz Hartmann, *Essays on Ego Psychology: Selected Problems in Psychoanalytic Theory,* The International Psycho-Analytical Library (London: The Hogarth Press, 1964; New York: International Universities Press, 1965), pp. 72 and 294.
12. Bernard Apfelbaum, "On Ego Psychology: a Critique," *International Journal of Psychoanalysis,* 47, pt. 4 (1966).
13. Clara Thompson, *Psycho-Analysis: Evolution and Development* (London's Allen and Unwin), p. 211.
14. Harry Stack Sullivan, *The Interpersonal Theory of Psychiatry* (New York: Norton, 1953), p. 21.
15. *Ibid.*

Chapter 3

THE
TURNING POINT:
FROM PSYCHOBIOLOGY
TO OBJECT-RELATIONS

HARRY STACK SULLIVAN
AND MELANIE KLEIN

Chapter 2 traced the struggle throughout Freud's work between the physicalistic type of scientific thought in which he had been trained and the need for a new type of psychodynamic thinking that he was destined to create. The first, or process theory, approach was enshrined in his instinct theory, which still persists even now in much of psychoanalytic terminology and writing: although his original quantitative theory of pleasure and unpleasure as physical processes determining all human action occurs now as no more than an occasional echo of the past. The second, or personal, approach became enshrined in his Oedipus complex theory, with its implications that it is what takes place between parents and children that primarily determines the way personality develops; and in his transference theory of treatment, that the object-relations of childhood have to be lived through again in therapeutic analysis if the patient is to grow from them. Only object-relational thinking can deal with the problem of meaning and motivation that determines the dealings of persons with another, and the way they change and grow in the process. The history of psychoanalysis is the history of the struggle for emancipation, and the slow emergence, of personal theory or object-relational thinking. Outside the confines of orthodox psychoanalysis and its organizations, early breakaway members pursued lines of thought that might have helped theory to move in this direction. Rank never became influential enough, and his contribution, as Ernest Jones shows, stimulated Freud but led to no particular goal. Adler certainly attempted an ego-psychology, but since he did little more, theoretically, than substitute the power drive for the early Freudian sex drive, Adler's theory simply swung from one extreme to the other; and since it also involved a swing from the unconscious to the conscious, it lacked the depth that was always so important in Freud's views. Sullivan acknowledged a debt to Freud, but unlike Adler's his thought was not mainly a reaction against Freud but a genuine development of his own independent insight. Sullivan's view that the biological substrate underpins, as it were, the life of interpersonal relationships, which is the real subject matter of the science of human beings, provides a sure theoretical basis for a properly psychodynamic science. In his own way Jung also transcended the biological for the personal, and developed an ego-psychology, a theory of individuation. Both Jung and Sullivan were men of unique intuitive powers. Freud was surely an unusual combination of the thinker who was both intuitive and systematic, and his great difficulty was that the systematic Freud felt obliged to build on what he had been taught, while the intuitive Freud went ahead to explore new paths. Yet he provided the beginnings of a systematic framework of theory, which however much it has proven to be necessary to change under the pressure of clinical experience, has proven equal to the strain of internal development and has in its own time taken into itself the insights of Sullivan and Jung. The steady psychoanalytical accumulation of clinical facts has at length brought its theory to the object-relational point of view, which the intuition of Jung and Sullivan, though in very different ways, jumped ahead to reach. It is the detailed psychoanalytical progress through about eighty years of research, to arrive at the present state of object-relations theory that I seek briefly to trace, through one or two of its main agents.

The work of Melanie Klein is the real turning point in psychoanalytical theory and therapy within the Freudian movement itself. Although Freud's own move into ego-analysis and group psychology beginning around 1920 prepared the way, there was something new in Klein's work. It is now a matter of history that a tremendous theoretical struggle raged in the British Psychoanalytical Society between the followers of Klein and the orthodox analysts who regarded her work as heresy. However it felt to those involved, it was a sign of vigorous intellectual activity. It cannot be dismissed as a purely internal affair because the issues were too important for the whole future thinking of psychoanalysis. Kleinians claimed and still claim that they are fundamentally orthodox and loyal to Freud. Apart from the fact that the idea of orthodoxy has no place in science, where there is no room for sects but only for the open-minded search for truth, we must also ask: "To which Freud? The physiological process theory Freud, or the personal object-relations theory Freud?" That question could hardly have been asked as long ago as 1930 in the way in which we are asking it today. Kleinians appeared orthodox enough, if that mattered in science, for they took over all of Freud's terminology of instinct theory, of id-drives of sex and aggression, and his structural scheme of id, ego, and superego, even outdoing most other analysts in orthodoxy to the extent of making the death instinct the absolute basis of their metapsychology. They simply claimed to be further developing Freud's thought in a logical way. Hanna Segal writes:

The Kleinian technique is psychoanalytical and strictly based on Freudian psychoanalytic concepts. The formal setting is the same as in classical Freudian psychoanalysis . . . in all essentials the psychoanalytical principles as laid down by Freud are adhered to.[1]

Yet their critics sensed that here was something new that seemed like a radical departure from the classical theory. And indeed there was, and it seems that Kleinians are themselves now realizing this as time has distanced the old controversy. Segal continues:

Could it be said therefore that there is no room for the term "Kleinian technique?" It seems to me that it is legitimate to speak of the technique as developed by Melanie Klein, in that the nature of the interpretations to the patient and the changes of emphasis in the analytical process show, in fact, a departure, or, as she saw it, an evolution from the classical interpretations. Melanie Klein saw aspects of material not seen before, and interpreting those aspects revealed further material which might otherwise not have been reached and which, in turn, dictated new interpretations seldom, if ever, used in the classical technique.[2]

That, I am sure, is correct, and I can see no reason why Melanie Klein's work should not be accepted as both an evolution and a departure from Freud's ideas. We expect evolution to produce something new.

I do not think that the apparently orthodox classical aspect of Kleinian theory, namely the perpetuation of the terminology of Freud's instinct theory, and his structural id-ego-superego scheme, along with his oral, anal, phallic, and genital concepts, is in reality as orthodox as it appears to be, though it

48

is more easily discerned now than it could have been at first. For one thing, there is very little of Freud's psychophysiological speculation surviving in Klein's work. She is without doubt psychodynamic. The only reason why we have come to make special use of the term object-relations as denoting a special type of theoretical emphasis, is that Freud, beginning his work in an age of material or natural science, took it for granted that the study of human nature in any scientific sense would *have* to be based on physiology and biology. It has taken a very long time to struggle through to the realization that that is a study of the *machinery* of the personal life, not of its *essential quality*, to use Freud's own term, a study of the mechanisms of behavior and not of the meaningful personal experience that is the essence of the personal self. Freud never really saw that in theoretical terms. Hartmann has followed him in this, and hopes that his system-ego theory "may prove capable of correlation with brain-physiology," and he wrote, "It is only when we consider the social phenomena of adaptation in their biological aspect that we can really start getting psychology rightfully placed in the hierarchy of science, namely as one of the biological sciences." The assumptions of Freud's early work are here persisting so strongly into his later work, that both Freud's and Hartmann's ego-theory remain tied to the ground and unable to develop to the level of a new psychodynamic science. This should stand firm in its own right as a scientific study of human beings, not as organisms, but as personal egos, whole selves in personal relationships, whose lives have meaning and value to them only in those terms. Melanie Klein's work is not at all a logical development of Freud's psychobiology in the way Hartmann's was.

Just how restrictive this tie to biology and ultimately physiology is, can be gauged from the fact that Hartmann's view of the function of the ego is that it is an organ of adaptation to be biologically understood. That is surely an utterly inadequate view of the ego, which psychologically is the core of self-hood in the person. *Adaptation* as the overriding aim ends up in the development of what Winnicott calls a "False Self" on a conformity basis. A "True Self" is not just adaptive but creative and able to contribute what is fresh and new to the environment. Even Erikson is restricted in his thought by this persistent undercurrent of thinking tied to biology and ultimately physiology. In *Childhood and Society* he writes, "I do not think that psychoanalysis can remain a workable system of enquiry without its basic biological formulations, much as they may need periodic reconsideration." [3] In his chapter, "The Theory of Infantile Sexuality," Erikson gives us just such a reconsideration, which as I hope to point out in the following chapter, wholly transcends biology in the sense in which Freud based psychoanalysis upon it. But it seems doubtful whether Erikson himself realized the extent of this, for the old id psychology dies hard. He writes:

The id Freud considered to be the oldest province of the mind . . . he held the young baby to be "all id" . . . the id is the deposition in us of the whole of evolutionary history. The id is everything that is left in our organization of the responses of the amoeba and the impulses of the ape . . . everything that would make us "mere creatures." The name "id" of course designates the assumption that the ego finds itself attached to this impersonal, this bestial layer, like the centaur to his equestrian underpinnings; only that the ego considers such a combination a danger.[4]

I find this passage astonishing and unrealistic, in its assumption that human nature is made up, by evolutionary "layering," of an ineradicable dualism of two mutually hostile elements. This would justify every pessimistic philosophy that human frustration and despair have ever thrown up. If it were true it would mean that the goal of a mature, whole human person is a fiction and is impossible. We would all be happier if we were frankly Centaurs, but in that case, though the "equestrian underpinnings" would remain bestial, the apparently human top half would not be truly human. The mythical figure of the Centaur is simply evidence of how far back in history human beings have suffered from pathological split-ego conditions. The use of this Centaur symbol as a model convinces me that Erikson did not see how effectively his own highly stimulating and insightful theory of zones, modes, and social modalities leaves biology and the id behind, and advances toward a consistently psychodynamic account of the ego as a whole person. It accounts for the fact that, in the end, I find Erikson's account of the ego tremendously enlightening as it is on questions of the social development of ego-identity, unsatisfying and lacking in fundamental depth. He writes:

Between the id and the super-ego, then, the ego dwells. Consistently balancing and warding off the extreme ways of the other two, the ego keeps tuned to the reality of the historical day . . . to safeguard itself the ego employs "defence mechanisms" . . . to arrive at compromises between id-impulses and super-ego compulsions.[5]

In his Foreword he writes:

Psychoanalysis today is implementing the study of the ego, a concept denoting man's capacity to unify his experience and his action in an adaptive manner . . . the study of the ego's roots in social organization.[6]

Erikson here lines up with Hartmann in falling back on the notion of adaptation, although more in a social than a biological context. In Chapter 5 we shall examine Hartmann's theory of adaptation in greater detail in contrast to the ego-development views of Winnicott. Freud's theory of the superego was in fact a study of the way in which the ego is influenced by social organization. There are other things in Erikson that involve a far greater emancipation from the classical biology than that, but I cannot accept his account of the ego attached to a dangerous impersonal bestial id as being adequate to human realities. It shows how tremendous has been the struggle to disentangle the two elements in Freud's original thought, the physiological and biological impersonal-process theory of id-drives and superego controls, and the personal object-relational thinking that has always been struggling to break free and move on to a new and more adequate conceptualization of human beings in their personal life.

It seems to me that, when we have disentangled the various conflicting elements in Melanie Klein's work, it becomes plain that it was Klein who, though unwittingly, made the great breakthrough. She had no choice but to start with Freud's psychobiological terms and to work with his unique clinical insights. These she developed, continuing to use his terminology, but her own clinical intuition, amounting to genius in her insight into the mental life of little children, broke through to explore new ground. As Segal claims, her work was both an evolution from Freud and a new departure, which called for some new terminology. It is important to clearly demarcate this new departure by comparison with the way others developed Freud's work. Hartmann continued the development of Freud's system-ego concept and remained frankly tied to biology. Erikson, just as consciously as Hartmann, set about the development of an ego-psychology, but along different lines, the "study of the ego's roots in social organization" and the delineation of ego-identities. This was clearly an object-relational study, yet he did not make as clear a break from psychobiology as Sullivan did, and so while having all the materials required, he still did not take the decisive step forward to a fully consistent psychodynamic account of human beings as whole-person egos. He still thinks in terms of an ineradicable internecine strife of structure, in which self-destruction is only avoided by the ego effecting compromises between the id and the superego. There is still no psychodynamic self or whole person. Where Hartmann extends classical psychoanalysis in the direction of general psychology, Erikson extends it in the direction of social anthropology.

Hartmann's tie to the id is at any rate consistent. I think that Erikson's tie to the id, "this impersonal bestial layer" as he calls it, is a radical inconsistency that prevents his theory from becoming a full genuinely personal psychology. Winnicott's research into ego-origins in the mother-infant relationship should have come first, and Erikson's study of ego-conditioning under cultural pressures could have followed logically afterward with greater effect. As it is, his ego-identities have no adequate psychic foundation other than the impossible bestial underpinnings of the Centaur.

But Melanie Klein did something essentially different from either Erikson or Hartmann, which is why I regard Melanie Klein's work as the decisive breakthrough in the development of psychodynamic object-relational thinking. She did not consciously aim at creating an ego-psychology, as Hartmann and Erikson did, and she appears to be every bit as tied to the id and the biology of instincts as Hartmann, and much more so than Erikson; especially when we consider the extraordinary way in which she treats the environment as a very secondary factor in the child's development, which Erikson would never have done. When Hartmann in his *Essays* speaks of "biological solipsism," perhaps he had Melanie Klein's views in mind. But it is just at this point that we sense a divergence from Freud. Freud's structural theory was based on the concepts of the control of instincts (the id) by the ego, under pressure from the external environment which led to the growth of the superego. Hartmann added to the ego the functions of adaptation, in conflict-free areas such as perception and motility etc., in the external world. Melanie Klein's structural theory developed in an entirely different way, eventuating in the concept of an internal psychic world of ego-object relationships.

Klein regarded an infant as an arena for an internal struggle between what at first were conceived of as the life and death instincts, sex and aggression, from the very start, quite apart from environmental influences. This ruthless inner drama then becomes projected onto the outer world, as the infant's brain and sensory organs develop the capacity to discern external objects. This means that the infant is never able to experience real objects in any truly objective way, and the way he does experience them depends more on his own innate make-up than on their real attitude and behavior to him. Basically, what he sees in his environment, is what he reads into it, mainly from his own internal terror of his own threatening death instinct. Segal tells us that "the death instinct is projected into the breast." This is then reintrojected, so that his experience of the outer world simply serves to magnify his impressions and double his anxieties on account of the internal dangers arising out of his permanently split nature. When Melanie Klein finally added an innate biologically determined constitutional envy to the infant's handicaps for any approach to reasonable and friendly objectivity in personal relationships, she seems to have left the environment with no real role to play at all. This makes her views appear to be so utterly incompatible with the outlook, not only of Sullivan, Horney, Fromm, and Clara Thompson but also of Erikson, Hartmann, and a whole range of American psychoanalysts, and no less incompatible with Fairbairn, Winnicott, and so many British analysts, that it is not surprising that it has aroused so much opposition. This has not been confined by any means to Anna Freud, Edward Glover, and the more avowedly classical analysts. If the environment plays such a minor and secondary role, it is little more than a mirror to reflect back to the baby its already existing internal conflicts. Hanna Segal explicitly says that the environment "confirms" (that is, it does not originate) the baby's primary anxieties and inner conflicts. It would seem then that such a theory could have little to contribute to object-relational thinking. There could be, one would think, no genuine object-relationships, when the objects-world seems to be of so little primary and intrinsic value.

Freud himself did not discount the environment in that way.

All this is true enough, but nevertheless it does not account for the whole of Melanie Klein's views. The more one surveys her theory as a whole, the more one gets the impression of a strange mixture of incompatible elements. One thing is clear that Melanie Klein explored much deeper into the mental life of tiny children than Freud had the opportunity to do. For this reason, she went beyond Freud's "father-dominated theory" and opened the way for the exploration of the mother's role in the baby's life. Furthermore, Melanie Klein did not take over Freud's instinct theory in the same way that Hartmann did. Hartmann made the distinction between what he called "Freud's clinical theory of sex and aggression" and his quite different "biological mysticism of Eros and Thanatos." Hartmann pursued Freud's clinical theory, although it is really more physiological than clinical, the theory of id-drives calling for an ego-control apparatus, and over and above that a system-ego operating its own techniques of adaptation to the outer world. Melanie Klein, on the other hand, took over Freud's biological mysticism of Eros and Thanatos, and saw human life as an intense hidden dramatic tragedy, a psychodynamic and fearful struggle between the forces of love and death inherent in the baby's constitutional make-up. Quite clearly, in Klein's estimation, the death instinct overshadows the love or life instinct, and is the true and ultimate source of persecutory and all other forms of anxiety.

This fundamental and innate conflict becomes observable, she held, in the infant's fantasy life as soon as it is developed enough to achieve clear expression, and we must remember that in clinical work with very small children, she found this internal fantasy world already well developed in children of between two and three years of age. This is not a matter of theory, but of verifiable, and now already verified, clinical fact, and it must begin to develop much earlier to be so complex by the fourth year of life. It is, moreover, an internal

world in which the child is living in fantasied and highly emo-
tion-laden relationships with a great variety of good and bad
objects that turn out ultimately to be mental images of parts
or aspects of parents. At the most primitive level they are
part-objects, breast or penis images, and later on they develop
into whole-objects that are in a variety of ways good or bad
in the infant's experience. *Life now is viewed, in this internal
world of fantasy and feeling, as a matter of ego-object relationships.* This may seem surprising in view of the fact that
the Kleinian metapsychology only allows a secondary role to
the external world. The infant can never experience the outer
world directly, but only through the medium of the projection of its own innate death instinct, and its fear of and struggle against it. These internal bad objects first come into being
as an introjection of the projected version of the infant's own
innate badness and destructiveness, and they have now become
worked up in its experience into parent images. Thus the external object world is forced on us again by the highly personal and psychodynamic nature of the infant's internal fantasy world. The fact is that, whatsoever the tortuous theoretical means, in Melanie Klein we find the term "ego" correlated
not now so much with the term "id" as in Hartmann and
Freud, but more and more with the term "object."

Klein's use of the term "id" appears to endorse Freud's instinct theory, but Freud's instincts do relate directly to external objects. Hanna Segal states, "Instincts are by definition
object-seeking," which had already been explicitly stated in
those words by Fairbairn (in order, however, to stress that
their aim was not pleasure, but the object that gives pleasure).
But in Kleinian metapsychology, instincts are lost in the dim
primitive mists of the mystic forces of Eros and Thanatos
warring inside the infant, irrespective of what goes on outside. They have, in fact, by making use of the outer world,
now become transmuted into internal objects. Kleinian instincts are primitive forces locked in combat inside the infant's

nature. The child's first love-object is its own primitive ego, in primary narcissism. Naturally, we have to remember that at birth there is no ego in a conscious sense, but there is a psychic self with ego-potential, out of which the sense of selfhood can gradually grow. For Klein, its entire psychic life is essentially bound up with itself, and out of this internal life consisting essentially of a hostile tension between two contradictory forces, a pattern world is created into which the child's experience of the external world is fitted. What seems to be by far the most important element in this solipsistic theory is that the child's first anxiety concerns its first hate-object. This is its own death instinct, which aims to bring about the organism's return to the inorganic state. The child could have no reason for projecting its love or life instinct, if such a phenomenon is conceivable. But if it is conceivable, it would most certainly have good reason to "project its death instinct," which threatens it with psychic destruction. It is only at this point that the Kleinian scheme finds it necessary to have an external environment into which this dangerous internal component can be extruded by the defensive illusion of projection. And now, the die is cast, the existence of external objects has been admitted and proven to be indispensable. They are indispensable because the infant is supposed to need them to project its death instinct into them, beginning with the mother's breast. But they are also inescapable, for they now constitute a real external threat that the infant has no real means of dealing with physically. It can only try to deal with it inside its own mental life again. The bad breast, now seen as containing a frightful destructive force, is introjected, and this death instinct now turns up inside no longer as an instinct but as an object, literally so perceived and fantasied. Because of her conception of the wholly internal origin of the active psychic life of the baby, Melanie Klein has to use external objects, and external object-relations, as a means of giving concrete expression to these theoretical primary forces and their hypothesized internal relations. What emerges as of first importance in all of this is not the more than dubious metapsychology of this biological mysticism but the way in which Klein brings to the front the highly important defensive procedures of projection and introjection that are certainly clinically verifiable facts; and then, of even greater importance, the fact that she has now interpreted the essence of the psychic life of the incipient person in fully ego-object relational terms. It is true that external objects are, apparently, valued not as objects in themselves but as receptacles for projection. However, the result comes to much the same thing in the end, namely the development of an inner world of fantasy that is actually object-relational, and is a counterpart of the ego's relations with the world of real objects that form its physical environment, centered in the mother. This is the real core of Melanie Klein's work. By a very devious and quite unnecessary theoretical route, based on hypotheses that hardly any other analysts but Kleinians accept, she arrived at the fundamental truth that human nature is object-relational in its very essence, at its innermost heart. This goes beyond all bio-physiological theories and is pure psychodynamics. Her much greater stress on projection and introjection in therapeutic analysis is a statement of the interaction of the two worlds, internal and external, in which all human beings live, so that finally the external world wins back the reality and importance that was denied it at the start.

Whereas Freud's theory was basically physiological and biological, I do not think that Klein's theory is in any genuine sense biological at all; it is philosophical, and more like a revealed religious belief than a scientific theory in its basic assumptions. Everything in life for Klein is dominated and overshadowed by the mighty and mysterious forces of life and death, creation and destruction, locked in perpetual struggle in the depths of our unconscious psychic experience, and constituting our very nature as persons. Of the two, it is the death instinct that steals the limelight all the time in Kleinian meta-psychology. Nevertheless, in therapeutic work, this theory facilitated the recognition of actual and new clinical facts. It is a highly psychodynamic theory, which led Melanie Klein to see and interpret in a peculiarly vivid way, the extraordinary extent to which infants, from the very beginning of postnatal life, develop in terms of the good and bad object-relationships that remain always associated, through projection and introjection, with the varieties of parental handling to which they are subjected. Her theory is confused because it inextricably blends the old and the new. Klein's original acceptance of Freud's theory seduced her into believing that her own insights were just a development of his views, and she perpetuated his biological terminology, thus distorting the significance of what she saw in her clinical experience. She claimed to trace Freud's Oedipus complex back into earlier ages than he himself had recognized. In truth she did something more important. Freud's Oedipus complex was itself the first clear expression of the fact that our adult personality operates over the top, so to speak, of a still surviving childhood life that centers in the conflicts of good and bad internal-object relations, in which the infant's first problems with parents, and especially the mother, become enshrined. Klein did trace this to a far deeper level than would have been possible for Freud to do, while he was struggling with creating the very beginnings of psychoanalysis. Her work was an evolution from, and also a departure from and a development beyond, Freud. What she really did was to display the internal psychic life of small children not as a seething cauldron of instincts or id-drives but as a highly personal inner world of ego-object relationships, finding expression in the child's fantasy-life in ways that were *felt* even before they could be *pictured* or *thought*. These could come to conscious expression in play and dreams, and be disguised in symptoms and in disturbed behavior-relations to real people in everyday living.

The study of the person-ego in object relations comes to be the real heart of Melanie Klein's work, however much it may be disguised by theories, many of which I for one find it quite impossible to accept.

The clearest proof that this is the really important thing in Klein's work can be shown by considering her treatment of the problem of stages of development. Freud's view of the stages of development was rigidly determined by the physio-biological factor of successive phases of instinct maturation, oral, anal, phallic (or preadolescent genital), and mature genital. Even so, Fairbairn regarded the anal phase as an artifact created by obsessive mothering, rather than a natural developmental phase. But these were all regarded as stages in the development of the sexual instinct. Libido was the basic sexual energy, and each of these organic zones was regarded as possessing its own inherent libidinal drive for the pleasure of de-tensioning. Infantile sexuality was oral, anal, or phallic; genital libido was mature or adult sexuality. As both Erikson and Fairbairn show, this is too simple and rigid to cover the real complex facts of individual development, although it was a valuable hypothesis as a starting point for investigation. This we shall consider further in the next chapter. For the moment we are concerned with Melanie Klein, and she on the face of it accepted Freud's scheme. All of us, of course, come across oral, anal, and genital clinical phenomena, and it would be odd indeed if the intense curiosity of the small child about everything in the complex fascinating world all around him did not also fasten on these highly obtrusive phenomena of his own bodily make-up, especially since they are so often apt to attract the wrong, disapproving kind of attention from anxious parents. But to recognize all this and the part that it plays in the emotional development of the personality is not the same thing as accepting Freud's theory that personality-development is dominated by a fixed timetable of biological instinctive maturational stages, oral, anal, and genital. Melanie Klein's pages are strewn with clinical observations of oral, anal, and genital material, and I would think that she was the first to make the highly important observation that children's sexual games do them no harm, provided that some disturbed child does not import aggression to the games.

When it comes, however, to the delineation of the stages of development, we find the center of interest shifting from the oral, anal, and genital scheme based on the idea of stages of instinct-maturation, and focusing on an entirely new scheme based on the idea of the quality of ego-experience in object-relations. This is a theory of two fundamental object-relational positions that the infant has to reach and adjust to in his emotional development *vis-à-vis* his mother in the first place, and thereafter in all personal relationships. Melanie Klein calls them positions because they are not just transitional stages through which the infant passes and grows out of and leaves completely behind. They are, in fact, a description of the two major problem positions in which the child finds himself as he tries to work out his relationships with the object world, beginning with the mother. Klein calls them the paranoid-schizoid position and the depressive position. She originally spoke only of the paranoid and the depressive positions, but later acknowledged specifically that Fairbairn's work had induced her to widen paranoid to paranoid-schizoid. It seems to me, however, that schizoid position is a third and separate concept. In the schizoid position the infant is withdrawn from object-relations. In the paranoid position, the infant is *in* relationship but feels persecuted by his objects. In the depressive position he has overcome these difficulties and has become able to enter more fully into whole-object relationships, only to be exposed to *guilt and depression* over the discovery that he can hurt those he has become capable of loving. We cannot regard these as three totally independent, clear-cut successive stages. There are overlaps and oscillations among all three of them. But in definitely bad mother-infant relationships, we must suppose that the infant will begin first to feel persecuted, then withdrawn into an attempted mental escape, then oscillating between these two reactions, and finally, if possible, growing beyond them to ambivalent relationships bringing guilt and depression.

Nothing more completely nonbiological and object-relational could be conceived, and it is a tremendous advance on Freud's scheme. Oral, anal, and genital phenomena now appear to be variations of symptoms, as emotional problems fasten onto one or another bodily organ to find bodily discharge in the conversion hysteria process. Klein's scheme is more fundamentally important than Erikson's highly interesting interpretation of Freud's scheme, in terms of modes of relationship rather than merely physical zones. I think, however, that both Klein's and Erikson's schemes are necessary, for Klein's scheme relates to the laying down of the basic possibilities of personal relationships within the first six months of life, and that determines how the child reacts in the more varied and incidental oral, anal, genital, and many other kinds of situations throughout the rest of childhood. Erikson's examination of all that appears to me to be of the highest value and to be fully object-relational. I have found these two schemes, taken together, along with Fairbairn's views of maturing from infantile dependence to adult dependence, form a valuable picture of the emotional vicissitudes that human beings encounter throughout life. They present a complex but fully object-relational schema.

Perhaps I have said enough to show why I regard Melanie Klein's work as constituting the decisive turning point in the emancipation of object-relational thinking from its imprisonment in the early classic psychobiology. I do not think she herself viewed her work in that way; that would hardly have been possible while she was in the thick of the struggle to clarify her new ideas. I do not think her present-day disciples see it that way, although they are aware that she did break new ground. Nevertheless, I believe this is how the history of psychoanalysis will finally see it, as the emergence of psychodynamic thinking out of physiodynamic thinking. As I have shown in Chapter 1, I am sure this is far more than just a domestic issue inside psychoanalysis. It involves the whole cultural and human problem of our age; that the study of human beings as persons involves science itself in moving into new territory where its traditional concepts and methods are no longer adequate, and a new area of scientific research comes into being, that of psychodynamics. The acceptance of this position must provide the intellectual basis for a more solid recognition of the rights of human beings as individual persons not to be "pushed around" by either scientific or political theorists, or educators.

In Freud, although his post-1920 ego-analysis prepared the way for a radically new orientation of psychoanalysis, object-relational thinking in his work remained to the end like a tethered race horse, there, but unable to run far from its starting post. In Melanie Klein, object-relational thinking is like a chained eagle, able to soar high above the ground even though it is still chained to it in her own thought. For Klein never intellectually questioned Freud's libido theory, as Erikson did, and thus never pursued the child's development in his social milieu as Erikson did. Nor did she radically question Freud's libido theory in the way Fairbairn did, and so did not make any special contribution to the ego-aspect of object-relations theory. As she presents them, her views appear to be a tremendous development of id psychology. Freud said that in many respects the superego is extremely close to the id, and in Klein's writing id and superego play a more important part than the ego. She did not develop any particular new trend in ego-conceptualization. In reality, however, while the infantile psyche is, for her, a secret arena in which Eros and Thanatos, the life instinct and the death instinct, are in unending warfare; in fact they are transmuted into a loving and creative ego and a hating and destructive, sadistic superego, an internalized parent as a bad object, imposing the pattern of their conflicts on perceptions of the outer world, in real-life object-relations. We can discard the biological and metapsychological or philosophical-mystical trappings of this theory, and recognize its clinical applicability as a fully psychodynamic and object-relational account of the internal development of the infant psyche. This clarifies all of the dangers of ego-splitting on the way to integrated maturity, as Fairbairn saw and worked out. But this psychodynamic view only becomes fully credible when it is interpreted in terms of the infant's developing relationship with his outer world, and his first significant object, namely his mother. That is what we find in the work of Winnicott.

We must add that only genuine clinical genius, manifested in extraordinarily direct intuitive insights, not only into adults but small children, could have enabled Melanie Klein to develop an essentially object-relational theory on the unpromising basis of apparently biological concepts. But clinical intuition is bound really to be object-relational, for it is a perception of what is going on in the immediate relationship of therapist and patient as two persons together, one of whom has to see correctly how they are relating in order to help the other to see, and so gain the chance to escape from the secret grip of infantile emotion and fantasy. This is what led Freud beyond his beloved neurology into the discovery of transference, Oedipal problems, and the formulation of the superego concept to clarify guilt feelings. It was that side of Freud's work that Klein developed. In spite of her verbal play with ideas of instincts, she was really concerned with good and bad object-relations, love and hate, and guilt and reparation, not with ideas of quantitative gratifications of instinctive drives. There could hardly be a more fully personal object-relational concept than reparation made for hurt of the loved person.

It is all this that leads to the most important element in what is called the technique of specifically Kleinian analysis. I shall discuss the use of this term "technique" of psychoanalysis in the final chapter of this book, but I am concerned here with the work of Klein, and her psychoanalytical method involves a greatly increased emphasis on the interpretation of the transference. For practical purposes, the essence of her work is to be found in (1) her theory of fantasy as the inner world life, which reveals itself as essentially an ego-function of relating to internal objects, good and bad (in spite of Susan Isaacs' explanation of it as the representative of instincts, a highly inadequate view), (2) her theory of stages of developmental positions, as clearly object-relational and psychodynamic, and (3) her increased stress on the use of transference in psychoanalytic therapy. We can be aware of how much her apparent classical orthodoxy and psychobiology hindered the free development of her object-relational thinking, but we do not have either to accept her whole or reject her entirely. Melanie Klein was one of the great creative minds of psychoanalysis, and we can recognize her highly original genius and make full use of her insights as marking a decisive turning point in the development of psychodynamic theory. The Kleinian psychoanalytic technique and psychotherapeutic use of transference is a good subject on which to close our examination of her contribution.

Transference is the phenomenon of the patient involving the therapist, who is part of his outer world, in the conflicts that constitute his inner world, and its analysis reveals the kind of interaction that is going on between his inner and his outer worlds, mainly by projection and introjection. To grasp the psychodynamic nature of Klein's inner world, we may contrast it with the inner world as conceived by Hartmann. For him, the inner world, "interposed between the receptors and the effectors," is simply the capacity to stop and think, to use intellectual judgment to avoid rash action. He is simply describing the psychic function of the intellect, which in fact has other and more creative uses in addition to signaling the red light and the yellow for caution, before it lights up the green for go. For Klein, however, the inner world is a far bigger thing. It is a whole object-relational private world of intense emotional experience, constantly competing with and interfering with our outer world living. Through transference-analysis the patient has the chance to become aware of how his two worlds of experience, inner and outer, are unrealistically confused, and he can slowly grow out of the resulting irrationalities of behavior. What I miss in Kleinian therapy, and what I think is ruled out by the nature of her theory, is any adequate recognition of the fact that analytical psychotherapy involves that the patient must grow out of unrealistic positive and negative transference relations, in which he is seeing his internal fantasied good and bad objects projected into his therapist, by means of discovering what kind of actual relationship is given to him by his therapist as a real person. This involves much more than experienced psychoanalytical interpretation. That paves the way, against the background of the kind of person the analyst actually is, for the patient to grow gradually to an accurate perception of him as a real person in his own right. For this to be possible, the analyst must be a whole real human being with the patient and not just a professional interpreter of the patient's psychic life. Only then can the patient find himself and become a person in his own right.

Melanie Klein's theory may be summed up thus: her inner world revealed in active fantasy as intensely object-relational makes up for the distinctly secondary place accorded to the outer world of real objects. In the strict logic of Kleinian views, the split personality of the infant expresses basically its constitutional nature in which its life or love instinct is permanently threatened by its death instinct (aggression, destructiveness, hate, and envy). This internal warfare must begin before birth, in the womb. It in no way reflects the infant's mixed good and bad experiences of external objects in real life. Klein is so occupied with the representations of these hypothetical instincts of fantasied internal good and bad objects that she more or less takes the ego for granted and does not develop any particular ego-psychology. This is the point at which Fairbairn's work develops. But the ego is there in Klein. With the formation of fantasy images, the child enters into his own fantasies and dreams as an ego relating to good and bad objects. For Klein, the origins of this fantasy life exist prior to the infant's experience of real objects, so that as his physical and mental perception of external real objects grows, he sees them through the colored medium of his already formed inner world, where he lives in terror of his death instinct. He does not have actual experience of mother as bad and then develop an internal bad object. He "projects the death instinct into the breast," according to Segal, and whether mother is bad or not, she is bound to be bad to the baby who sees her as carrying his own innate badness. Bad-object experience is overwhelmingly primary for Klein who has then to say that the baby urgently needs to internalize a good breast to counteract it. I cannot see how, on Klein's assumptions, a baby can ever experience a really good breast at all. Even if he does (by projecting his love instinct, which we hear little about), the death instinct must always ruin it. Theoretically, the problem is insoluble because bad-object experience for Klein is primary and ineradicable. In actual therapeutic analysis, however, no doubt the real personal relationship of analyst and patient is more important than theory. What we have in Klein is acute clinical perceptiveness, distorted by preconceived theory. If we leave out the speculative theory, mostly centered on the death instinct, we are left with the foundations of object-relations theory firmly laid in clinical analysis of the inner world fantasy life, and the transference reactions of the patient to the analyst.

NOTES

1. Hanna Segal, "Melanie Klein's Technique," *Los Angeles Psychoanalytic Forum* 2, no. 3 (1967): 198.

2. *Ibid.*, p. 199.

3. Erik H. Erikson, *Childhood and Society*, rev. ed. (New York: W. W. Norton; London: The Hogarth Press, 1964), p. 64.

4. *Ibid.*, p. 186.

5. *Ibid.*, p. 187.

6. *Ibid.*, p. 13.

7. Hanna Segal, *Introduction to the Work of Melanie Klein* (London: Heinemann Medical Books, Ltd., 1964), p. 12.

Chapter 4

THE BROADENING
THEORETICAL
REORIENTATION

ERIK H. ERIKSON AND
W. RONALD D. FAIRBAIRN
≡≡≡

I have been dealing with the subject of object-relations theory as the gradual emergence to the forefront of the personal as against the impersonal, or natural science, element in Freud's thought. It is the story of the slow evolution of a new type of scientific thinking, namely psychodynamics. This key to the whole process was recognized by Erikson, when in 1955 he reviewed Freud's letters to Wilhelm Fliess, published as *The Origins of Psychoanalysis*. Erikson commented on the emergence of "a radically new kind of intellectual process, specific for psychoanalytic work and thought." [1] I have regarded Melanie Klein as the important turning point in theory, because she does, although in a confused way, present a major change of emphasis away from organically determined processes, and toward the concentration of attention on psychodynamic object-relations. Freud, working largely alone,

69

thirty to forty years earlier, and necessarily in the dark as to the goal he would arrive at, could not possibly have clarified at once, and then consistently held fast to "the radically new kind of intellectual process, specific for psychoanalytic work and thought" that was slowly growing in his researches. Those who have the advantage of being able to look back at a battle after it is over can see more clearly even than the general who was in charge just what was going on during it, even though, had they been in his place, they would not have had the ability to fight and win it. It is easy for us now to forget the entrenched intellectual prejudices in the scientific world of Freud's early days, in which he could not help but share, and so fail to understand how slow and difficult his progress was bound to be. The extraordinary thing is that he, and he alone, set out to explore this new pathway of thought.

Even forty years later it was difficult for most of those who had dared to follow Freud, to see clearly what it was that was really new. Melanie Klein, certainly at first, regarded her work primarily as simply tracing conflicts of instincts back to a much earlier level in infancy than Freud had the chance to do. Freud himself never clearly distinguished and properly related the physiobiological and the personal object-relations' elements in his thinking. His last and unfinished book, *The Outline of Psychoanalysis,* provides fascinating evidence of how near and yet how far Freud was to solving this problem of letting psychodynamics stand on its own feet as a new scientific development. On the first page he writes:

We know two things concerning what we call our psyche or mental life: firstly, its bodily organ and scene of action, the brain (or nervous system), and secondly our acts of consciousness, which are immediate data and cannot be more fully explained by any kind of description. Everything that lies between these two terminal points is unknown to us and, so far as we are aware, there is no direct relation between them. If it existed, it would at the most afford an exact localization of the processes of consciousness and would give us no help towards understanding them.[2]

The inference, surely from this entirely clear and adequate statement, is that we must leave the brain and nervous system to physiology, which will provide the knowledge needed to deal with physical problems arising in the biological substrate, but cannot be looked to, to cast any light at all on our subjective living as persons. This indicates the need for the creation of a new scientific discipline, namely psychodynamics. But Freud still feels this must remain tied to physical science. He continues:

Our two hypotheses start out from these two ends or beginnings of our knowledge. The first is concerned with localization. We assume that mental life is the function of an apparatus to which we ascribe the characteristics of being extended in space and of being made up of several portions—which we imagine, that is, as being like a telescope or microscope or something of that sort. The consistent carrying through of a conception of this kind is a scientific novelty.[3]

Again, surely, that is exactly what it is not. It is an attempt to form a conception of mental life on the basis of a physical model, and that after he has already said that physical processes can "give us no help towards understanding" mental processes. In psychology we are not concerned with localization (that is the concern of physiology), rather our concern is with meaning and motivation and purpose. But Freud goes on to deal with our psychic life on his physical telescope model, "extended in space . . . and made up of several portions." He speaks of it as a "psychical apparatus" with "mental provinces."

To the oldest of these mental provinces or agencies we give the name of *id*. It contains everything that is inherited, that is present at birth, that is fixed in the constitution—above all therefore the instincts. . . . Under the influence of the real external world which surrounds us, one portion of the id has undergone a special development. From what was originally a cortical layer . . . a special organization has arisen which henceforth acts as an intermediary between the id and the external world. This region of our mental life has been given the name *ego*.[4]

The mixing rather than the relating of two different types of concepts is clear. Are these aspects of our psychic or mental life, provinces or agencies? A province is a spatial area, a material reality. An agency is the expression of a free and active purpose, a psychic reality. Freud tells us that the ego has the tasks of "control of voluntary movement. It has the task of self-preservation" by means of "becoming aware . . . storing up experiences . . . flight . . . adaptation, and, finally, by learning to bring about appropriate modifications in the external world to its own advantage (through activity) . . . (and) by gaining control over the demands of instincts." [5] We have passed, without an admission of the fact, from a "province extended in space" to an "active mental agent with complicated purposes." Yet Freud still seeks to tie these to physiology.

Its activities are governed by consideration of the tensions produced by stimuli present within it or introduced into it. The raising of these tensions is in general felt as *unpleasure* and their lowering as *pleasure*. . . . The ego pursues pleasure and seeks to avoid unpleasure.[6]

We are now back at square one. After the promise of a real psychodynamic science, with the recognition of "our acts of consciousness which are immediate data" that have "no direct relation" to the brain and nervous system, and if they had, such knowledge of physical localization "would give us no help toward understanding them," we are plunged right back into the original physiological tensions of the pleasure principle, or quantity principle. This is confirmed when Freud writes:

The forces which we assume to exist behind the tensions caused by the needs of the id are called *instincts*. They represent the somatic demands upon mental life. . . . After long doubts and vacillations we have decided to assume the existence of only two basic instincts, *Eros* and the *destructive instinct*.[7]

This is where Freud finished his work. When he wrote those words, he was nearing the end of his life and one could not expect anything other than a reaffirmation of what basically he had always held to. Yet even so, the last unfinished chapter suggests that had Freud been able to renew his youth and start again where he left off, he would not have stopped at this point. After accounting for the superego as the result of the parent's influence on the child, an object-relational not a biological fact, his last words were, "In the emergence of the superego we have before us, as it were, an example of the way in which the present is changed into the past." [8] He had already explained this by saying the superego "unites in itself the influences of the present and the past." Here are experiences that can only be understood as "acts of consciousness," experiences of our personal relationships, about which brain physiology can tell us nothing, and that still remain after all to be understood as realities in their own right. Freud created psychodynamics, as Erikson says, "a radically new type of scientific thinking, specific for psychoanalytic work and thought," without clearly differentiating it from physical science.

It will not surprise us then to have found the same mixed thinking in the work of Melanie Klein, although in fact her analysis of the inner psychic life back to earliest infancy in terms of ego-object relations was a development of the personal element in Freud's thought, and carries us far beyond Freud's psychobiological starting point, and also far beyond the position in which he finished up in his last statement. Joan Riviere, one of Klein's closest collaborators, quoted Anna Freud on the autoerotic and narcissistic infant "governed by the desire for instinctual gratification, in which perception of the object is only slowly achieved." Riviere comments, "Here (Anna Freud) makes a distinction between 'object-relations in its proper sense' and the 'crudest beginnings of object-relations built up in the initial stage.' There can be no such distinction since the 'beginnings' are the object-relations appropriate and proper to the earliest stage of development."[9] Kleinians were led to discard Freud's primary objectless phase.

We may now look at the work of Erikson and Fairbairn as illustrating in very different ways how an increasing reorientation of theory from the impersonal to the personal object-relations basis proceeded, after Klein. Since there is strictly speaking no object without an ego to perceive and relate to it, it is more complete and meaningful to speak of ego-object relations theory, and this brings out the fact that from now on we become ever more concerned with the meaning, nature, and growth of the ego, as the impersonal id fades in significance. Freud was deeply concerned with the ego from 1920 onward, but to the last, in *The Outline*, the ego is still only a partial affair, a province or agent mediating between the id and outer world up to the age of about five, by which time the ego has taken part of the outer world into itself, that is, the parents who observe it, give orders, correct and punish it, to create a new psychic agency, the superego.[10] The ego is not really the I, the core of selfhood in the person. Freud takes the whole self for granted and nowhere discusses it specifically as the one psychic phenomenon that matters most of all. A perusal of the index of his collected works shows that Freud discusses self-analysis, self-preservation, self-punishment, self-esteem, self-regard, self-reproach, and so on, but never *The* Self as the unique individual person. Ego-psychology broadened considerably with the work of Harry Stack Sullivan, Karen Horney, Erich Fromm, and Clara Thompson, without, however, reaching its full significance. Their work, however, prepared the ground for Erikson's ego-identity studies. Sullivan brought the term "self" into prominence but only gave it the same kind of partial and limited meaning that Freud allowed it. He spoke of the "self-system" or "self-dynamism" as a culturally determined anxiety product. "The self-dynamism is built up out of the experience of approbation and disapprobation, of reward and punishment. . . . The self may be said to be made up of reflected appraisals." [11] So limited is the ego in Sullivan's view, that he actually says, "As it develops it becomes more and more related to a microscope in its function. . . . It permits a minute focus on those performances of the child which are a cause of approbation or disapprobation, but, very much like a microscope, it interferes with noticing the rest of the world. . . . The rest of the personality gets along outside of awareness." [12] This is not the basis for a whole-person-ego psychology. It only answers to what Winnicott would call "a false self on a conformity basis" and offers us no help for a psychology of "the true self." It is interesting that Freud and Sullivan both independently used the idea of a microscope to stand for the psychic apparatus or the self. We need a different approach, but must first proceed from the Sullivan school to Erikson, and then to Fairbairn. Dates are significant here for tracing development. Melanie Klein began to publish papers in 1920, and her first book appeared in 1932. Fairbairn's published papers began to show the influence of Klein from 1933 and by 1940, he had found his own individual line. Fairbairn's highly original papers of the 1940s appeared in book form in 1952. Erikson's first book had appeared in 1950 but that also was the fruit of long prior experience. Thus Erikson's and Fairbairn's dates run roughly parallel in their earlier work and first book, although Fairbairn published in the Journals ten years before Erikson. Melanie Klein antedates both of them by up to twenty years.

I deal with Erikson first because, although his work is far wider ranging sociologically, it is not as radical psychodynamically as Fairbairn's. In his 1955 review Erikson stated uncompromisingly the full extent to which Freud's work was rooted in "Physicalistic physiology. The ideology of this important movement was represented in Du-Bois-Raymond's and Brücke's oath—'No other forces than the common physical ones are active within the organism.' " [13] Concerning Freud's *Psychology for Neurologists* in 1895, Erikson says Freud aimed "to see how the theory of mental functioning takes shape if quantitative considerations are introduced into it." [14] The clear inference is that since Freud abandoned this work, he found it impossible to formulate psychoanalysis as a natural science. Erikson records how hard a struggle Freud had in order to make the transition. He writes of the Fliess letters as giving a "vivid picture of him in the difficult years during which his interest shifted from physiology and neurology to psychology and psychopathology." He describes Freud as being "daemonically obsessed with the inner necessity to reconcile the ideology of his past discipleship in physiology and his now unavoidably approaching mastership in psychology." [15]

Thus, there can be no doubt that Erikson was entirely clear as to the magnitude of the issue at stake. Does he think that Freud really did outgrow his past? He writes of Freud defending himself against his anxieties by a "grandiose persistence in the physiological ways of looking for well-differentiated tissues, pathways and lesions." On the other hand, Erikson describes Freud's *Dream Book* as a "complete and systematic breakthrough to the rich mines of symbolism and inner dynamics which set Freud free"; free to "lead consciousness into psychomythology and clinical psychology," and to psychoanalysis as "a radically new kind of intellectual process." It is wholly true that this was a genuine breakthrough into real psychodynamics, but it is not wholly true that this set Freud free from his past. The old and the new lived on side by side. Erikson finally writes of Freud's "creative misconceptions—a persistence which disposes of traditional assumptions not by abandoning them, but by pursuing them to the bitter end, where radically new assumptions emerge." [16] In fact, as the final *Outline of Psychoanalysis* showed, the radically new assumptions did emerge and found Freud still retaining the old ones at the same time. Actually in *The Outline* the old assumptions are more in evidence than the new ones.

We must turn to a seldom-quoted work of Freud to realize the acute problems this created for him in the practical matter of treating patients by analysis, and how courageously he brought the new elements in his work to the very front place. In 1926 he published *The Question of Lay Analysis*. The question arose because in Austria the law prohibited anyone who was not medically qualified from treating the sick. Freud was uncompromising. He stated that in the matter of neurosis, "patients are not like other patients," and that, provided the person who treats the neurotic is properly trained in psychoanalysis, "laymen are not, properly speaking, laymen, and physicians not precisely what one is entitled to expect in this connection." [17] Going more fully into this Freud writes:

The medical profession has no historical claim to a monoply in analysis. . . . A quack is a person who undertakes a treatment without possessing the knowledge and capacity required for it. On the basis of this definition, I make bold to assert that doctors furnish the largest contingent of quacks in analysis—and not only in European countries. They very often use analytical treatment, without having learnt it and without understanding it.[18]

What he is really struggling with, apart from the practical problems of treatment, is the fact that a training in physical science is useless for understanding the working of the mental personality. This has far-reaching implications for both therapy and theory. Freud is entirely clear as to therapy. After making it plain that medical examination and diagnosis must first establish whether the patient's trouble is really emotional and not physical, that is, the doctor must rule out organic causes, and when physical symptoms arise during the course of analysis, the patient must be referred back to the doctor to make sure physical factors are not primarily involved, he then makes an uncompromising statement, to the effect that a training in physical science is far from being the best one for understanding human beings in their personal life.

The analytical curriculum would include subjects which are far removed from medicine and which a doctor would never require in his practice; the history of civilization, mythology, the psychology of religion, and literature. Unless he is well-orientated in these fields the analyst will be unable to bring understanding to bear upon much of his material. And, vice versa, he can find no use for the greater part of what is taught in medical schools. A knowledge of the anatomy of the metatarsal bones, of the properties of carbo-hydrates, of the courses of the cranial nerves, of all that medicine has discovered as to bacillary infection and means to prevent it, or neoplasms—all this is of the greatest value in itself, but will take him nowhere. It will not directly help him to understand and cure a neurosis, nor does this sort of knowledge sharpen the intellectual faculties on which his professional activity will make such demands. The analyst's experience lies in another field from that of (physio)pathology, with other phenomena and other laws.[19]

My concern in quoting from this monograph is to show how absolutely clear Freud was, when the practical problems of treatment were concerned, that he had indeed broken into a new field of scientific research, involving "a radically new kind of intellectual process." (Erikson) It is startling to find that the man who in 1895 could aim at "a psychology which shall be a natural science," could in 1926 write the following:

In the medical schools the student's course of instruction is more or less the opposite of what he would need as a preparation for psychoanalysis. His attention is directed to objective, verifiable facts of anatomy, physics and chemistry. . . . The problem of life is brought into consideration, in so far as it has emerged, up

to now, from the play of forces which are demonstrable in inorganic matter also. No interest is evoked in the psychological
side of vital phenomena; the study of the higher achievements of
the mind is nothing to do with medicine. . . . Psychiatry alone
is concerned with the disturbances of mental functioning but one
knows in what way and with what purposes? Psychiatry looks for
the physical causes of mental disorders and treats them like those
of any other illness. . . . Psycho-analysis, indeed, is particularly
one-sided, being the science of the unconscious mind. So we need
not deny to medicine the right to be one-sided. . . . But medical
training does nothing towards either evaluating "the neurotic's"
case or treating it—absolutely nothing. . . . The situation would
not be intolerable if medical training simply denied to doctors any
approach to the field of neurosis. But it does more; it gives them a
false and positively harmful attitude towards it. Doctors, having
had no interest aroused in the psychical factors in life, are all too
ready to disparage them.[20]

It must be said, in all fairness, that far more psychiatrists today
than in 1926 are looking for an understanding about psychical, and not just physical cause of emotional illness. But
there are many psychiatrists and medical men about whom
Freud's words are as true now as they were when they were
written. While I was lecturing in New York, one of my patients in England had an acute anxiety-attack and was rushed
into a mental hospital. When she was discharged, she was told
that all possible physical tests had been made, that all the find-
ings were negative, and there was absolutely nothing wrong
with her. Such a pronouncement simply could not have been
made by anybody who had had an adequate knowledge of her
abnormally sad life-history. One can understand Freud closing
his argument with these words:

We do not want to see psychoanalysis swallowed up by medicine,
and·then to find its last resting-place in textbooks on psychiatry—
in the chapter headed "Therapy," next to procedures such as hypnotic suggestion, auto-suggestion, and persuasion, which were
created out of our ignorance, and owe their short-lived effec-

79

tiveness to the laziness and cowardice of the mass of mankind. . . . As "psychology of the depths," the theory of the unconscious mind, it may become indispensable to all the branches of knowledge having to do with the origins and history of human culture and its great institutions; such as art, religion and the social order.[21]

I know of no more trenchant statement of the fact that psychoanalysis has broken into a new field of phenomena as far as science is concerned, and "a radically new kind of intellectual process, specific for psychoanalytic work and thought" is needed. I would merely observe that today psychoanalysis can no longer be defined as "the theory of the unconscious mind." It has become the theory of the whole person, of the personal ego in personal object-relations, good and bad, growing either mature or basically disturbed.

In view of Freud's absolute distinction between training in the physical and psychodynamic science, his concern that training restricted to physical science can blunt a student's comprehension of psychological facts and even prejudice them against the acceptance of psychic realities as facts in their own right, and his view that he does not want psychoanalysis to be swallowed up in medicine, that is, in physical science, one would expect to find Freud as definite and uncompromising in his distinction between psychoanalysis as the psychodynamic science of our subjective life as persons in relationships, and physical or natural science as the sciences of the material basis and setting of our personal life. But here Freud wavers, and as we have seen he was unable to the very end to make that clear-cut distinction in theory that he made so absolutely in practice. I can agree, therefore, that Freud's "creative misconceptions" were pursued "to that bitter end where radically new assumptions emerged," but I also feel that Erikson underestimates the extent to which Freud's failure to "abandon the traditional assumptions" led to his "disposing" of them. In fact the old and the new continued mixed and confused. It was Freud's failure to abandon the traditional assumptions of science, not of course in their proper natural science sphere, but in this new sphere of the psychodynamic study of human beings as persons in their meaningful individual lives, that led to the confused and illegitimate mixture of biology and psychodynamics, which has so seriously delayed intellectual clarification in this field. Jones, Kris, and Erikson all maintained that Freud did transcend physiology for psychology. I suspect that they believed this because they did not fully transcend physiobiology and arrive at a full consistent psychodynamics themselves. Like Freud, they superimposed psychology on top of biology, which is not the same thing. The truth is that Freud and his progressive successors both did and did not transcend natural science. The "radically new kind of intellectual process," which is psychoanalysis, does not deal with quantity but with quality, value, meaning, and motivation in the personal self. How absurd it would be to try to explain or understand such concepts as maturity and love in quantitative terms. Psychoanalysts in general have not made Sullivan's clear distinction between the biological substrate as one level of abstraction in studying the psychosomatic whole human being, and subjective personal experience and interpersonal relations as an equally real but quite different and higher level of abstraction in studying human reality. Even K. M. Colby, who was clear about this, ends by giving us a mechanistic model of personality structure.

Thus, as we saw in the last chapter, Erikson allows physiology and biology to be carried along by the new psychology. This is why instinct theory, a purely biological view of sex and aggression, and the id concept, still appear as fundamental in writers whose original work has moved beyond such ideas. In 1951 Joachim Flescher of New York even suggested a hypothetical organic substance, which he proposed to call aggressin, as a physical basis for aggression, so as to get in the same instinct-basis as sex. It is better to eschew such hypothetical speculation and simply accept sex as an appetitive ego-reaction and aggression as a defensive emotional ego-reaction, which is simply a factual clinical statement. Fairbairn was the one analyst who saw entirely clearly this problem of mixing and confusing different disciplines, and made a definite break with it. The effects of not making a clean break are visible in Erikson's work. His deeply interesting Chapter 2 of *Childhood and Society* on "The Theory of Infantile Sexuality" goes a long way beyond the classical instinct theory. Erikson regards the term "instinct" as being more applicable to animal than to human psychology. He writes, "The drives man is born with are not instincts; nor are his mother's complementary drives entirely instinctive in nature. Neither carry in themselves the pattern of completion . . . ; tradition and conscience must organize them." [22] Again, "as an animal man is nothing. . . . Man's 'inborn instincts' are drive fragments to be assembled, given meaning and organized during a long childhood. . . . The vague *instinctual* (sexual and aggressive) forces which energize instinctive patterns in man . . . are highly mobile and extraordinarily plastic." [23] It is a measure of the difficulty of making a clean break with an over-familiar terminology that has outlived its usefulness, that in repudiating instinct-theory Erikson still falls back on using instinct terminology, speaking of "the vague instinctual (sexual and aggressive) forces" even though he has already said, "The drives man is born with are not instincts." The view of Gordon W. Allport, although still not fully satisfactory, seems somewhat in advance of Erikson here. He writes:

The doctrine of drive is a rather crude biological conception . . . inadequate to account for adult motivation, useful to portray the motives of young children. . . . After infancy primitive segmental drive rapidly recedes in importance, being supplanted by the more sophisticated type of motives characteristic of the mature personality.[24]

Erikson and Allport both accept the idea of infantile organic drives that are later woven into culturally determined adult motive-patterns. I do not regard that as satisfactory because it perpetuates the idea of the personality as a psychosocial pattern developed later on the foundation of purely biological drives at the beginning. There cannot be any time when a human being is all soma and no psyche. Psyche and soma are there together from the most primitive or early stage to the latest and most developed.

In that sense Freud was extraordinarily perceptive in his day to trace sexuality back to infancy, although it would probably be less confusing to use the term "sex" for the specifically genital, and the term "sensuous" for the important "bodily contact needs" of the infant for maternal handling, accepting that somatic stimuli can flow into the sexual genital organs in earliest infancy, without, however, having the same significance as it will have at a later age. Concerning the so-called instinct of aggression, Allport stated, "Aggression is not a primary tendency to hurt or destroy, but an intensified form of self-assertion and self-expression . . . a secondary result of thwarting and interference." [25] That is Erikson's view. He writes of:

That second primeval power, the assumption of which followed the concept of the libido in the psychoanalytic system . . . an instinct of destruction, of death. . . . I shall not be able to discuss this problem here, because it is essentially a philosophical one, based on Freud's original commitment to a mythology of primeval instincts. Freud's nomenclature and the discussion that ensued have blurred the *clinical* study of a force which will be seen to pervade much of our material *without* finding essential clarification; the *rage* which is aroused whenever action vital to the individual's sense of mastery is prevented or inhibited.[26]

Aggression is a defensive reaction of a threatened ego. Erikson has discarded Freud's biological mysticism and makes aggression analyzable as "a reaction of intensified self-assertion in face of thwarting," according to Allport, a thwarting of "the individual's sense of mastery." It is thus not an id-reaction but an ego-reaction. Erikson here abandons the id-concept and thinks only in terms of ego-experiences.

In his handling of infantile sexuality, Erikson actually takes up the same position without clearly stating it. He treats it as a complex of ego-reactions, not as an id-drive. In what he writes about the id, Erikson clings illogically to a theory he has in fact abandoned: a view of human personality as constructed of layers, primitive and biological at the beginning; cultural, social, sophisticated, and psychological at the top, id and ego. This I believe to be a false view, which needs to be superseded by a view of the psyche-soma as a whole that does not have primitive survivals inside it, but a whole in which everything that is taken up into it is transformed in a way that makes it appropriate to its being part of this whole. This view is not invalidated by the existence of a few biological vestigial features, since by definition they are now of no active importance. This is the view really implied in Erikson's theory of infantile sexuality. He does not work with the idea of a specific quantity of instinctual libidinal drives constitutionally inherent in the oral, anal, and genital zones. His scheme of zones, modes, and social modalities is different in principle. The organism has its place in the bodily zones (oral, anal, genital), but also in all the other organs (hands, eyes, ears, and skin). The psyche has its place in the modes of object-relating, which can be associated with any or all of these zones. The social environment has its place in those relatively stable ways of relating that become built-in parts of the social cultural mores. His scheme states the basic ways in which an individual can relate to an external environment, particularly with respect to persons. They are limited in number, but they find expression equally in both the mental attitudes of the individual and in the bodily organs he possesses, since he relates as whole entity with mind and body at the same time.

Erikson is not afraid to use the term "mind" without implying dualism. He writes:

> In recent years we have come to the conclusion that a neurosis is psycho- *and* somatic-, *and* social-, and *inter*personal. . . . These new definitions are only different ways of combining such separate concepts as psyche and soma, individual and group . . . : we retain at least the semantic assumption that the mind is a "thing" separate from the body.[27]

> We are speaking of three processes, the somatic process, the ego process, and the societal process (which) have belonged to three different scientific disciplines—biology, psychology and the social sciences—each of which studied what it could isolate. . . . Unfortunately this knowledge is tied to the conditions under which it was secured: the organism undergoing dissection, the mind surrendering to interrogation, social aggregates spread out on statistical tables. In all of these cases a scientific discipline prejudiced the matter under observation by actively *dissolving its total living situation* . . . to make an isolated section of it amenable to a set of instruments or concepts. . . . We study individual human crises by becoming therapeutically involved in them . . . and find that *the three processes mentioned are three aspects of one process— i.e., human life,* both words being equally emphasized. Somatic tension, individual anxiety, and group panic, are then only different ways in which human anxiety presents itself to different methods of investigation.[28]

This is a splendid, robust, critical refusal to allow separate scientific disciplines to dictate to our clinical thinking, on the basis of their study of only partial aspects of the psychosomatic whole self, or person-ego. Erikson accepts Sullivan's view of the biological substrate and goes on to deal with human life as a total process of interpersonal relations. Erikson writes, "Terminological alignment with the more objective sciences . . . should not keep the psychoanalytic method from being what Sullivan called 'participant.' The same applies to psychoanalytic theory. If it is to be meaningful about what is its true subject of study, it must relate to the 'whole person.' " [29]

One aspect of this calls for closer examination. Given the body, the mind-ego, and society as three separate fields of study, and accepting Erikson's work on the way in which particular patterns of ego-identity are shaped by social, environmental influence that can be seen to be ever more influential as the individual grows older, yet the relationship between the mind-ego and the body is quite different from that between the mind-ego and society. The mind-ego depends existentially on its body in a way it does not so depend on society. But this apparently complete dependence and "being at one with" does not obliterate the distinction between the body and the mind-ego. As far as we know, the mind-ego depends for its existence, totally on the body, but it depends on society, the human environment in particular beginning with the mother, for its chance to develop its full ego-potential. Here psychodynamics goes beyond Freudian psychobiology in which the body is the source of powerful id-drives that dictate to a weak and superficial ego. I regard this view of a human being as made up of evolutionary layers, in which dangerous unmodified survivals of the primitive past trouble the present as quite unacceptable. In psychodynamic science the opposite view is being worked out. The body, accepted as the biological substrate and foundation of the mental or personal life, has become part of a greater whole in such a way that the actual functioning of the body is determined in enormously complex ways by the personal life it sustains. It is naive to think of a primitive id dictating to a socialized ego, or *vice versa*. We must think of a psychosomatic whole person, in whom the fate of the organism is far more complexly determined by the psychic self in humans than in animals, because the psychic self of humans is far more complex than is that of animals. Leaving aside mental deficiency resulting from brain damage and similar problems, we have the whole scale of phenomena ranging from all the proliferating psychosomatic diseases, through the hysteric and particularly conversion hysteric illnesses in which the psychic self or mind-ego can avoid direct recognition of its problems by, so to speak, pushing them into the body, right up to the psychosomatic wholeness of the mature person, where the life of the body is healthily exercised and invigorated, without being abused, by the spontaneous enjoyment of living in the inwardly anxiety-free person. The body would not be the same kind of body and would not function in the same way if it were part of a different psychic whole. It has been assumed hitherto that mind (that which enabled the scientist to create his science) was a kind of secretion, if anything, of the body. But we now have to think in terms of a developing psyche as the vital stimulating factor evolving a body to meet its needs. The psychic self or mind-ego uses the body both for symbolic self-expression and for direct action, and for both together as a psychosomatic whole, not as a poor little defensive ego at the mercy of powerful id-drives or organic instincts. The stimulus of Freud's work, which was so original in the early years of this century, has led quite properly to its own supersession, as far as much of the theory is concerned.

This seems to me to be the concept implied in Erikson's reinterpretation of Freud's oral, anal, and genital scheme of development. To Erikson, the terms oral, anal, and genital, represent orifices or zones of the body that are material modes or ways of relating to objects. These become developed in different cultures into recognized social modalities or ways of carrying on human relations. The mental attitude and the use of a bodily zone belong together, making up the response of a whole person to his world. It is not a case of libidinal organs with fixed drives such as oral libido, anal libido, and genital libido, governing behavior. As Fairbairn pointed out, the self can both libidinize and delibidinize behavioral organs. The modes or ways of relating represented by body zones are equally and at the same time represented by mental attitudes having the same significance. Moreover, the striking thing about Erikson's scheme is that each body zone does not stand exclusively for what is generally regarded as its own characteristic mode; every zone can use all the modes. Erikson writes; "The functioning of any orificial body zone requires the presence of all the modes as auxilliary modes." [30] For a baby or simple organism, all ways of relating to objects can be reduced to a small number of possibilities and these remain the basic ways of relating all through life. These ways are basically four, but since two of them can function in two different ways, they are basically six, namely getting, keeping, invading: but getting may be either peaceful reception or angry seizing, and giving out may be either a true giving or a rejection, a throwing away. Thus there are six basic ways of relating, receiving, grabbing, keeping, giving out, rejecting, invading, or attacking. These can be loosely associated with but are not identical with Freud's oral, anal, and genital reactions.

The two ways of getting—peaceful receiving and angry seizing—are clearly expressed in Freud's two oral incorporative modes, oral sucking and later on oral biting. For Erikson the mouth has no monopoly on these ways of relating. The infant's whole mental attitude of needing to get and take in, is expressed in other ways as well. Erikson writes:

To the infant, the oral zone is only the focus of a first and general mode of approach, namely incorporation. . . . He is soon able to "take in" with his eyes what enters his visual field . . . His tactile senses seem to take in what feels good. [31]

The infant opens and closes his hands on objects and conveys them to his mouth. He needs not only to take in orally but to "find pleasure in being held, warmed, smiled at, talked to, rocked, etc." In fact he "takes in" with his entire body and mind. The expression of the first need to get and incorporate from the environment in order to live may focus on the mouth, but is not expressed only by the mouth. The whole psychosomatic person, both bodily and mentally, expresses this need. The mouth can also employ modes that seem to belong to other zones. It can also spit out and reject, and retain and hold on, like the anus, and it can attack or invade, and seek to burrow into the breast like a penis, or bite its way into food, or even bite as a form of fighting, as do animals and occasionally humans.

Thus we are led on from oral incorporation to the anal zone, with its two modes of retention and elimination. Anal retention may express anxiety or the fear of losing, as well as anger, stubborn resistance, refusal to give out any latent aggression. Elimination is of two kinds, an effortless letting go, which may express love, a free giving out to the mother of what she wants but also an angry casting out, rejecting. Freud called this term anal hate, the classic term for dirtying. The five modes of relating to objects that focus on oral and anal zones but express the purposes of the whole infant person include taking in, seizing, holding on, giving out, and angry rejecting. These represent the mental attitudes that can be expressed not only through one particular body-organ, but in a variety of kinds of behavior. Lastly, we come to the genital zone, which in certain ways further develops the incorporate mode of the oral zone in the female, for taking in remains a permanently necessary mode of relating to the outer world. Clearly, it must depend on the whole personality whether this genital "taking in" in a woman is a masochistic suffering of invasion, or sadistic seizing, or a loving receptivity. One female patient could never have orgasm until her husband had withdrawn, for she actually felt that her vagina was a hungry mouth that might harm him. In the male, the genital zone is characterized by what Erikson calls the "intrusive mode," which is invading and exploring, but in an aggressive male it will be sadistic, in a mature loving male giving. As the infant must begin by taking the world into himself, so he must become able to go out into his world and enter into its life and relationships, bodily and mentally. Erikson's term "intrusive mode" is not the happiest one to describe this process. It has a slight bias toward aggression, but he uses it to describe the infant's progress from "being done to" to active "doing." He writes:

The *intrusive* mode dominates much of the behaviour of this stage, and characterizes a variety of "similar" activities and phantasies. These include the intrusion into other people's bodies by physical attack; the intrusion into other people's ears and minds by aggressive talking, the intrusion into space by vigorous locomotion: the intrusion into the unknown by consuming curiosity.[32]

It is clear that while this mode includes aggression, it is not in essence aggressive, but rather self-assertive, the expression of the growing small child's need to feel his own reality by finding that he can make an impact on his environment, and deal actively with it.

By using the term "intrusive" (that is, forcing a way in uninvited), Erikson risks suggesting that male sexuality is essentially aggressive, a relic of the days when classical analysts talked of sadistic and masochistic instincts. But, in reality, we are very far here from Freud's psychobiological libido theory. We have arrived at a properly psychodynamic description of the manifold means by which a human infant develops the fundamentally possible ways of relating, as a vigorously growing psychosomatic whole person, to his mother, family, and the outside world. Erikson has converted Freud's libido theory into an object-relations theory. We see the emerging person-ego growing, at first most obviously by the use of his material body to deal with his material environment, taking in what he needs (air, food, water, warmth, contact) and being receptive to needed mental and emotional stimuli; rejecting what he does not like or want (feces, urine, undigested food, food that he finds not nice, dropping and throwing away objects, turning away from people whose atmosphere is not right, not reassuring), learning gradually to join with, cooperate, and work with those who care for him to achieve his ends (with mouth, hands, ears, eyes, legs, and whole body, and growing understanding), all the time in ways that are oral, anal, genital, and also mental, and becoming increasingly personal. There is nothing here about the seething cauldron of Rapaport's id-drives in the unconscious, which are a danger to both the ego and the environment. What we have is a detailed account of how the infant gets to know and live with his object-world, and to develop an ego. After giving us this realistic account, I find it disappointing that Erikson still finds room for the highly unrealistic Centaur model of the supposed human id-ego. The implications of this absurd comparison are that we would all be mentally healthier if we were Centaurs (since Centaurs are not so troubled by their dual nature as humans are). This is not a theory that helps us to understand human nature, but a vivid warning of the dangers of allowing biology to hang on to the developing psychodynamic object-relations theory. The danger is clear when Erikson writes, "Psychoanalysis studies the conflict between the mature and the infantile, the up-to-date and the archaic layers of the mind." The equation of "mature" with "up-to-date" and "infantile" with "archaic" is a misleading error perpetuated by the idea of evolutionary layers of the psychosomatic whole. It needs to be replaced by the concept of an evolutionary whole in which every constituent is appropriately different from what it would have been in a different kind of whole.

It is here that I turn with relief to Fairbairn, who clearly saw this problem of making theory consistent. He totally rejected the id concept. It appears to me that its origins (in Groddeck) could well be analyzed as a conversion hysteria symptom-concept, an intellectualized attempt to project the needy, frustrated, angry life-urge of the infant, out of the psychic self or personal ego into some impersonal nature beyond and outside the ego or real I. Once invented, the id concept has stuck, but it appears as if Freud was trapped in the problems of his self-analysis when he accepted Groddeck's "It," and saw the poor little ego struggling between the vast impersonal forces of the id and the pressures of society. Fairbairn started by rejecting Freud's divorce of energy and structure (a point Colby arrived at ten years later) as a survival of outdated Helmholtzian physics. Instead of a primitive id, all untamed energy, and a weak, energyless structural ego, he saw the human being, not as built up of layers like a brick wall, but as a psychosomatic whole. Thus Fairbairn wrote:

Impulses cannot be considered apart from either object or ego-structures. Impulses are but the dynamic aspect of endopsychic structures, and cannot be said to exist in the absence of such structures. Ultimately "impulses" must be regarded simply as constituting the forms of activity in which the life of ego-structure consists.[33]

Recognizing that energy and structure do not exist apart, that we no longer think in terms of the billiard-ball universe where energy moved solid atoms around in space, and regarding energy and structure as aspects of the same whole enabled Fairbairn to work with the concept of a whole human being from the very beginning of life, normally whole at every stage from the most primitive to the most developed. The baby starts life as a whole psychic self however primitive and undeveloped and undifferentiated. Fairbairn writes, "The pristine personality of the child consists of a unitary dynamic ego." [34] What Joan Riviere said of object-relations, Fairbairn could say of the ego, that the crudest beginnings of ego-feeling developed in the initial stage are the ego-feeling appropriate and proper to that earliest stage of development. He rejected the view that the ego is a later synthetic growth. The human psyche, simply because it is human, contains the innate potentiality of ego-growth in a way that the animal psyche does not. The psycho-somatic whole of the human being does not begin as a bestial layer of animal instincts blindly seeking detensioning, so that the trained social environment has to conjure up a controlling ego "on the surface of the id," whatever that may mean. The human infant is a unitary dynamic whole with ego-potential as its essential quality from the start. In the late nineteenth century the concept of the person did not exist philosophically in the way it does today, as the concept of an irreducible reality, and individuality *per se*. "Person" is not the same as "Personality." Personality is either an emphatic term for the unique force or quality of some particular individual, or more generally in psychology it is only a pattern or configuration of characteristics, such as that which psychologists make inventories of. Person is the essence of the truly human being at every level of development. Freud did not start with the concept of the whole person. Psychoanalysis became obsessed with distinguishable aspects of psychic functioning as parts needing to be fitted together, as in Glover's ego-nuclei theory where separate bits of ego-experience fuse into an ego. That is why the name "psychoanalysis" has persisted, a name appropriate enough to the investigation of a material object, but not very appropriate to the sympathetic healing study of a person whose wholeness is in jeopardy.

Fairbairn believed that we must be primarily aware of the fundamental dynamic wholeness of the human being as a person, which is the most important natural human characteristic. To Fairbairn the preservation and growth of this wholeness constitutes mental health. The question of primary importance from birth onward is not the gratification or satisfaction of instincts, not the control of impulses or drives, not the coordination or reconciliation of independent psychic structures, all of which arise because of the loss of the "pristine unitary

93

wholeness of the psyche." The question of first importance is the preservation, or if lost, the restoration of psychic wholeness, the safeguarding of the basic natural dynamic unity of the psyche developing its ego-potential as a true personal self. Mental illness is the loss of this basic natural unity of the ego. *Mental health* is its preservation from disintegration in passing through the maturational stages on the way to adult maturity. *Psychotherapy* is the reintegration of the split-ego, the restoration of its lost wholeness. I have heard the criticism that Fairbairn and I envisage a disembodied psyche, ignoring biology, a psyche without a soma. That is a total misconception. Fairbairn regarded the human being as a psychosomatic whole, not a psyche-soma dualism, not a Centaur. But he clearly saw that just as biology studies the somatic processes by methods that throw no direct light on our subjective personal experiences, so psychodynamic science studies the subjective personal experiences of the psychosomatic whole person by methods that throw no direct light on biological processes. He opposed the intellectual confusion of mixed disciplines.

This comes out clearly in Fairbairn's theory of libido. Classically, libido is a quantitative energy permanently attached to bodily zones. Fairbairn discarded libido as a biological entity or force *per se* as involving the error of reification of some element or aspect of a complex whole process. He spoke, therefore, of the libidinal ego, which can libidinize any part of the body it wants to use for making a relationship, not just mouth, anus, genitals; but skin, muscles, eyes, ears, and hands just as Erikson described. I have a patient, who whenever he suffers a mild separation anxiety, not only libidinizes his mouth so that saliva flows and he feels a craving to eat, but at the same time he gets hay fever as he calls it, which libidinizes his nose so that it flows, causing him to rush to swallow antihistamine tablets. One session of analysis or even a telephone conversation is now sufficient to relieve both libidinizations, because contact has been restored and his separation anxiety has died down. At other times when he feels withdrawn, he can delibidinize both mouth and nose, which become dry. This is a clue to the nature of conversion hysteria symptoms, which represent repressed good or bad object-relationships experienced in the body: leading on one hand to over-stimulated sexuality, on the other hand to impotence, frigidity, or physically painful symptoms, bodily masochism. Fairbairn treated sexual problems as hysteric conversion symptoms, that is, as internal bad-object-relationships with either the exciting object or the rejecting object. Thus we deal not with a permanently localized biological entity called the libido, but with a person, a libidinal ego who can libidinize or delibidinize any part or the whole of the body according as he feels intense need for, or withdrawal from, human intimacy. For Fairbairn, "the goal of the libidinal ego is the object," and libido is a technical term for the basic object-seeking life-drive of the human psychic self.

The entire process of growth, disturbance, and restoration of wholeness as an ego or personal self depends upon the ego's relations with objects, primarily in infancy, and thereafter in the unconscious (the repressed infantile ego split and in conflict) interacting with object-relations in real life; not just any objects, material things, toys, foods, but the all-important class of objects who are themselves egos, human objects beginning with the mother, and proceeding if necessary to the psychotherapist. Once the mother is possessed by the baby, she can be represented symbolically by things, cuddly toys, what Winnicott calls transitional objects, on the way toward developing a less exclusively mother-centered need, as long as the first all-important human object, the mother, remains reliable enough. At first it is the mother who is herself a healthy whole ego who enables the baby to perceive and develop his own wholeness as an ego. Whole ego development depends on good object-relations in real life, either initially in infancy or later on in therapy. Split ego development arises out of bad object-relations in real life. Here Fairbairn disagrees radically with Melanie Klein. For Klein the baby is split from the start by nature, a battleground of life and death instincts. Bad-object fantasies basically represent the threat of the death instinct and this is its original experience, so that Melanie Klein naturally holds that the first object to be internalized must be the good object, the good breast, if the infant is to have any chance of stability. Two comments seem necessary. First, it is difficult to see how the infant can internalize a good breast, since he is supposed to project his death instinct into the breast and re-introject that, now as a bad internal object. As I showed in the last chapter, it is this that converts Klein's theory from an instinct-theory into an object-relations theory. Second, it is after all the bad-object that is first internalized, for the infant could have no reason to project its life instinct. Kleinians tend to deny that they give only secondary value to real external objects, but I do not think they can legitimately make that claim. Their basic theory forbids it. This is quite clear from the following quotations from Hanna Segal's *Introduction to the Work of Melanie Klein*.

The immature ego of the infant is exposed from birth to the anxiety stirred up by the inborn polarity of instincts—the immediate conflict between the life instinct and the death instinct. . . . As the death instinct is projected outwards, to ward off the anxiety aroused by containing it, so the libido is also projected, in order to create an object which will satisfy the ego's instinctive craving for the preservation of life.[35]

Thus it is the reintrojection of projected instincts that creates objects in the psychologically meaningful sense, and it *is* the bad-object that is introjected first, as Fairbairn held, because it is the death instinct that is projected first and reintrojected first.

The importance of the environmental factor can only be correctly evaluated in relation to what it means in terms of the infant's own instincts and phantasies. . . . An actual bad experience *confirms* . . . his feeling that the external world is bad.[36]

Fairbairn rejected that view totally. The infant is by nature whole and would remain so if protected long enough by good-object relationships in his dealings with the real world, and primarily the mother. Good object experience simply leads to good ego development. A proof of this is surely the fact that there are people who have had good enough mothering and have grown up with adequately stable and mature personalities. However, perfection in fact being impossible, the infant soon encounters unsatisfying parental experience, and it is the bad-object mother in real life who is first internalized in an effort to control her. Since she is not wholly bad, the unsatisfying mother, after internalization, is split into a good mother and a bad mother; and usually the good mother is projected back into the real external mother who is then idealized so as to make real life relations as comfortable as possible. One patient started analysis by saying "I have the most wonderful mother on earth," which immediately made me realize that her mother was her real problem, as turned out to be the case. The good object serves as a protection against the bad object externally, but internally the bad object is a threat to the good object, because of the hate aroused. Thus an internal situation of fear of harming the good object results, with feelings of guilt and depression. The bad object is itself split as an internal object into an exciting object and a rejecting object. The exciting object is then incessantly longed for, setting up the compulsive and emotional needs always found in chronic dependencies, and, in an attempt to control this situation, which there is no real way of relieving, the rejecting object is identified with, and a sadistic superego, or to use Fairbairn's own highly appropriate term, an antilibidinal ego grows out of identification with the parent who refuses to meet the child's needs.

This splitting of the object in the struggle to cope with unhappy real life experience leads to a splitting of the ego in the struggle to maintain relations with both the good and bad aspects of the mother and other family figures. Fairbairn reduces Klein's multiplicity of internal objects to three basic fantasied figures who can appear in many guises: (1) the tantalizing mother who excites needs without satisfying them, *the exciting object;* (2) the rejective, angry, authoritarian, antilibidinal mother who actively denies satisfaction, a mild form being the mother who says "Don't bother me now, I'm busy," *the rejecting object;* and (3) the emotionally neutral, morally idealized mother whom the child seeks to view without much feeling, with whom needs are avoided so as to avoid her displeasure, and with whom conformity is accepted in hope of at least approval, the ideal object. The exciting and rejecting objects are both bad and are repressed as twin foci of a troubled unconscious emotional inner world. The ideal object is projected back into the real parent in the hope of living at peace in the outer world. With this object-splitting goes a parallel ego-splitting: (1) an *infantile libidinal ego* unceasingly stimulated by the exciting object, hungrily craving the personal relations without which the psyche cannot grow a strong ego, but manifesting in adult life as chronic overdependency, compulsive sexuality, and craving for appreciation; (2) an *infantile antilibidinal ego* identified with the rejecting object, an undeveloped childish conscience, negative and hostile, self-persecuting, inducing fear and guilt, the main source of resistance to psychotherapy; (3) a *central ego* conforming with the idealized parents, after the emotionally disturbing aspects of both objects and ego have been split off and repressed. This seems to me the most accurate theoretical analysis I have come across, of the pattern of the split-psyche that underlies psychoneurosis and psychosis.

I cite here a concrete expression of this in dream form. One male patient in his forties dreamed: "I was sitting up against a wall and both the wall and I myself were cut in two parts, an upper and a lower part, above and below my waist, with a gap in between." His immediate comment was, "I came in with my eyes smarting as if I could burst into tears (he had shed tears for the first time in the previous session and felt more real and whole afterward). I feel emotional, but I'm trying to think things out, to think of something to say, I think—no, I've lost it. There's nothing now." I interpreted, "You feel split into a thinking head above, and a feeling abdomen below (which can turn over or feel butterflies when you're emotionally moved.) And now you've fallen into the gap between them. There's nothing, but in fact you are directly experiencing your split self. You are in the process of overcoming this and bringing your thinking self (that is, the central ego) and your feeling self (that is, libidinal and antilibidinal egos) together." How real the split between the parts of the self in the unconscious, tied to bad parental-objects, whether merely exciting or rejective, can be, is shown in two experiences of another male patient, both brought out in the same session. (1) He had grown his hair very long, and people were commenting on this, but he said, "I like to look at it in the glass. It excites me sexually," and then went on to say that people often told him that he looked like his mother in appearance. She had in fact been emotionally exciting to him in his earlier childhood and had become increasingly authoritarian and rejective as he grew older, once angrily pushing him into the street and locking him out. In growing his hair long and looking like his mother, and feeling excited as he looked into the mirror, he was actually expressing concretely his feeling that he possessed his exciting object inside himself, and yet never felt satisfied. I put this to him, and he went off on another topic. (2) He said, "I'm not anti-racial, and this sounds artificial, but all this weekend I've been angrily talking to a group of immigrants who have an authoritarian religion, are strict with their children, and who form an enclave in our society, refusing to be integrated. At any rate that's what I'm feeling about them." I said, "This sounds to me like the other side of your mother, not the exciting one but the strict, bossy one, who locked you out, and whom you dream of as stealing your car, your penis, and making you impotent. She's an enclave in your make-up and refuses to be integrated, but crushes your spontaneity." Here was his internal rejecting object.

These splitting processes begin certainly as soon as the mother's primary maternalism (vide Winnicott) begins to fail the baby. The resulting loss of unified experience of both objects and self continues to ramify and complicate every stage of later development. Fairbairn dismisses the anal stage as an artifact dependent on obsessional mothers. Instead of oral, anal, and genital stages, he reinterprets oral, anal, and genital psychopathology as conversion hysteria; he suggests a different scheme of developmental stages based upon object-relations experience: (1) *immature dependency* (infancy), (2) *a transitional stage* (latency and adolescence), and (3) *mature dependence* (arrival at adult capacity for full and equal personal relations). Fairbairn regards the world of internalized objects as coming into being in the first stage of infantile dependence and persisting thereafter as the psychopathological unconscious. He accepted Klein's two basic developmental positions, paranoid and depressive, as belonging to this earliest infantile period, representing the two internal bad-object situations in which the infant can be trapped. But he regarded schizoid as being not an aspect of an inevitable developmental position but a fear-dictated flight from object-relations, the deepest root of mental illness. If the depressive position is central, as Klein maintained, for moral development, the schizoid position is the fundamental one for the loss or preservation of that ego-wholeness that is the basis of mental health.

Erikson's reinterpretation of oral, anal, and genital phenomena, as not necessarily psychopathological, but as natural parallel bodily active zones and mental modes of object-relating, fits easily into this over-all view, as giving important developmental details. It seems to me that a combination of Klein, Erikson, and Fairbairn gives us a very thorough overall view of the details and problems of early human development. I think we must concede to Fairbairn recognition as the one psychoanalytic thinker, who, over twenty-five years ago, unequivocally stressed object-relations experience as the determining factor, the all-important desideratum, for ego-development, the required form of psychoanalytic theory. His work, however, as far as the ego goes, stopped at the analysis of ego-splitting, and still leaves open the final problem, that of the origins of the ego, to which we shall turn in the next chapter.

NOTES

1. Erik H. Erikson, "Freud's The Origin of Psychoanalysis," *International Journal of Psychoanalysis*, 36, pt. 1 (1955): 1.
2. Sigmund Freud, *The Outline of Psychoanalysis*, ed. and trans. James Strachey (London: The Hogarth Press; New York: W. W. Norton, 1949), p. 1.
3. *Ibid.*, p. 1.
4. *Ibid.*, p. 2.
5. *Ibid.*, pp. 2–3.
6. *Ibid.*, p. 3.
7. *Ibid.*, p. 5.
8. *Ibid.*, last chapter.
9. Joan Riviere, in Melanie Klein et al, *Developments in Psychoanalysis* (London: The Hogarth Press; New York: Hillary House, 1952), p. 12.
10. Freud, *The Outline*, p. 77.
11. Harry Stack Sullivan, *The Interpersonal Theory of Psychiatry*, eds. Helen S. Perry and Mary L. Gawel (New York: W. W. Norton; London: The Hogarth Press, 1968), pp. 20–22.
12. *Ibid.*
13. Erikson, "Freud's The Outline of Psychoanalysis."
14. *Ibid.*
15. *Ibid.*
16. *Ibid.*
17. Sigmund Freud, *The Question of Lay Analysis* (London: Imago Publishing Co., 1947), p. 2.

18. *Ibid.*
19. *Ibid.*, p. 77.
20. *Ibid.*, pp. 58–59.
21. *Ibid.*, p. 79.
22. Erik H. Erikson, *Childhood and Society*, rev. ed. (New York: W. W. Norton, 1964), p. 89.
23. *Ibid.*, pp. 89–90.
24. Gordon W. Allport, *Personality: A Psychological Interpretation* (London: Constable, 1949).
25. *Ibid.*
26. Erikson, *Childhood and Society*, pp. 62–63.
27. *Ibid.*, p. 19.
28. *Ibid.*, pp. 32–33.
29. *Ibid.*
30. *Ibid.*
31. *Ibid.*, p. 66.
32. *Ibid.*
33. W. Ronald D. Fairbairn, *An Object-Relations Theory of the Personality* (New York: Basic Books, 1954), p. 88.
34. W. Ronald D. Fairbairn, "Observations on the Nature of Hysterical States." *British Journal of Medical Psychology*, 27, pt. 3 (1954): 105–125.
35. Hanna Segal, *Introduction to the Work of Melanie Klein* (New York: Basic Books, 1964), p. 12.
36. *Ibid.*, p. 4.

Chapter 5

THE CRUCIAL ISSUE:
SYSTEM-EGO
OR PERSON-EGO

HEINZ HARTMANN,
DONALD W. WINNICOTT,
AND EDITH JACOBSON

═══════

We must now summarize our argument and show how biology and psychodynamics must be both distinguished and properly related, instead of mixed and confused. Then psychoanalysis can attend to its own proper business, studying the unique individual person growing in the medium of interpersonal relations. I shall do this by comparing some aspects of the views of Heinz Hartmann, Donald W. Winnicott, and Edith Jacobson. The title of Winnicott's 1967 volume, *The Maturational Processes and the Facilitating Environment*, related biology and psychodynamics in an essentially object-relational way. The maturational processes are the biological given, the innate constitutional potentialities continuously unfolding as the individual lives. They presuppose an individual whose potentialities they are. He does not live *in vacuo* but rather in an environment. His innate potentials do not mature willy-nilly in sublime indifference to his outer world. They require an environment that understands, supports, and permits individual growth. If the environment does not satisfy these needs, development will be both arrested and distorted. The true self, which is latently there, is not realized. A false self emerges on the pattern of conformity or adaptation to, or else rebellion against, the unsatisfactory environment. Its aim is survival in minimum discomfort, not full vigorous spontaneous creative selfhood. The result is either tame goodness or criminality. The individual whose nature contains latent maturational processes requires a facilitating environment in which to grow, and this is first and foremost the infant's own mother if a healthy, stable, cooperative, and creative person is to emerge. The implications of this will become clear by contrast with Hartmann's view of psychoanalysis as a biological science. Jacobson's position is, in some respects, between these two and contains elements of both viewpoints.

The title of Hartmann's 1937 essay was *Ego Psychology and the Problem of Adaptation*. "Adaptation" was his key word. It belongs to biology. He wrote: "The foundation on which Freud built his theory of neurosis was not 'specifically human' but 'generally biological' so that for us the difference between animal and man is relative." [1] One would think that the fact that animals cannot be psychoanalyzed implies that psychoanalysis is a specifically human discipline to be distinguished from generally biological studies. Hartmann did not draw that inference. He stated, "An investigation such as this one, which uses man's relation to his environment as its point of departure, should focus on action." [2] By relation, he means not personal relation but activity-relation, the biological behavioral viewpoint. A psychopersonal viewpoint would focus on experience rather than on action, on being prior to doing. For Hartmann, man is an adapting organism, not an intrinsically meaningful existent having absolute, not relative value, in de-

veloping forms of unique individuality that will never be re-
peated. He writes, "We call a man well-adapted if his productivity, his ability to enjoy life, and his mental equilibrium are
undisturbed . . . and we ascribe failure to lack of adaptation.
But degree of adaptiveness can only be determined with reference to environmental conditions. The conception of adaptation has no precise definition. It was long cherished by biology
. . . but recently has been frequently criticized and rejected."
But Hartmann was not warned by the limitations of this concept even in biology and proceeded to apply it in psychology,
simply saying, "Psychoanalysis alone cannot solve the problem
of adaptation. It is a subject of research for biology and sociology also." [3]

Psychoanalysis began with a defective realization of the importance of the concept "Person," owing to the cultural era
of its origin. Thus Freud could take the term "id" from Groddeck, who wrote, "We should not say 'I live' but 'I am lived
by the It.' " This completely destroys the unique and responsible individuality of the person. It reflects the materialistic
determinism of the nineteenth- and early twentieth-century
science. Hartmann refers to this "id" as "the personality's central sphere" beyond which lie "other realms of mental life."
They include the autonomously developing apparatuses, techniques, preconscious automatisms, and regulating principles of
the ego, which he defines as "an organ of adaptation." The
first business of the ego was to prevent Groddeck's "It" from
"living us" willy-nilly, and compelling it to bow to the need for
adaptation to the environment. Hartmann extended ego-theory
as a general psychology, showing that not all ego-processes
are developed out of conflict with id-drives, but grow autonomously with reference not to the id but to the outer world.
Apparatuses of perception, thinking, object-comprehension,
intention, language, recall-phenomena, productivity, motor-
development (grasping, crawling, and walking), maturation,
and learning processes generally developed outside the area

of conflict, in what he called the "conflict-free ego sphere." [4] Granted the id-theory, this needed to be done. He distinguished between "Ego-functions involved in conflicts with the id and superego, and ego-functions concerned with coming to terms with the environment." [5] Thus Hartmann's theory is rooted on the one hand in the biological id, and on the other hand in the equally biological concept of "adaptation." His ego has two aspects: it is an organ of defense against the inner world, and an organ of adaptation to the outer world.

Like Freud, Hartmann writes of two kinds of adaptation, *autoplastic*, or altering oneself to fit in with the environment, and *alloplastic*, or altering the environment to fit in with oneself. He comments, "Neither is necessarily truly adaptive. A high ego-function must decide what is appropriate." [6] But this goes beyond biology and admits more than the theory will bear. What do "truly adaptive" and "appropriately adaptive" mean? What is this "higher ego-function"? Is it merely practical judgment as to what adaptation will or will not secure organic survival, or is it an entirely different evaluating function expressing the higher values of the true self? In that case the ego must be more than just an organ of adaptation. This would aim not at physical survival but at preserving the integrity of the person and the defense of his values. Hartmann's biological theory does not properly admit of this second possibility. On the properly biological level there is little chance of genuine alloplastic adaptation. The animal lacks the intelligence and means to alter his environment except in such small ways as are better called making use of what is there rather than making the environment different to fit into its own needs. Being incapable of using the science and technology of man, the animal has to adapt to its natural environment or perish as many species have done. Thus the age of the reptiles, the dinosaurs, and brontosaurs lasted about 200 million years and then completely disappeared, even though it included the tyrannosaurus, which is supposed to have been the most powerful land-dweller of all time. On the other hand, if adaptation is sufficiently successful, it results in stagnation. There are species so well adapted that they have remained unchanged and static for millions of years. A turtle exists today whose bones are exactly the same as those of a turtle that existed long before the dinosaur. The real meaning of biological adaptation is fitting in to the environment for the sake of survival. The more the concept of "adaptation" is varied and sophisticated beyond that basic simple meaning, the further it gets from biology. By the time we have defined adaptation in terms of a human being and his environment mutually adapting to each other, we are far beyond biology, and we must go further still. The concept of the environment has now changed. It no longer means nature in general. Science enables us to cope with that for most practical purposes. The part of the human environment that is most significant is the society of his fellow human beings. A human being may have to refuse to adapt to his human environment, and he prepares to lose his life in order to save something that is more precious to him than biological survival, his "soul," his truth to himself as an individual who means something that is of intrinsic value. To talk of the ego as an organ of adaptation in that context is simply irrelevant.

In studying human living, "adaptation" is replaced by a higher concept, that of a *meaningful relationship* in terms of values. Hartmann almost saw that when he said that neither autoplastic or alloplastic adaptation "is necessarily truly adaptive." What I think ought to be said is that neither is necessarily truly significant for interpersonal relationships. Adaptation can be raised to the level of personal relationships, but personal relationship cannot be reduced to the level of adaptation. If I am convinced that someone is more right than I am on some issue, I can change my view and accept his, or I can be prepared to cooperate with someone I love to do something that would not otherwise interest me. This may be seen as autoplastic adaptation raised to the level of personal relationship. Alloplastic adaptation, forcing other people to alter to fit in with us, is totally debarred from interpersonal relations. We call it totalitarianism. We may use persuasion and win their assent, but that rises again to the level of interpersonal relations. When Hartmann wrote, "A higher ego-function must decide what is appropriate" or "truly adaptive," it would be truer to say, a higher concept of the Ego than that of "an organ of adaptation" is necessary, to understand interpersonal relations. Adaptation, strictly speaking, can only express one-sided fitting in. Personal relations involve mutual self-fulfillment in communication and shared experience, of two or more people. Hartmann is, of course, aware of the complexity of the problem of what he calls adaptation, when it moves from the animal to the human level. He writes:

What is the structure of the external world to which the human organism adapts. . . . We cannot separate the biological from the social conditions. The first social relations for the child are crucial for the maintenance of his biological equilibrium also. It is for this reason that man's first object-relations became our main concern in psychoanalysis. Thus the task of man to adapt to man is present from the very beginning of life. . . . Man adapts to an environment part of which, has not, but part of which has already, been moulded by his kind and himself. The crucial adaptation man has to make is to the social structure and his collaboration in building it. We may describe the fact that the social structure determines, at least in part, the adaptive chances of a particular form of behaviour, by the term *social compliance* coined in analogy to "somatic compliance" which is implied by the concept of adaptation . . . By adaptation we do not mean only passive submission to the goals of society but also active collaboration on them and attempts to change them. The degree of a person's adaptation is the basis of the concept of health.[7]

This very significant passage shows the serious confusion of thought that is inevitable when biological and personal are not clearly differentiated, when the distinctively human is allowed to be absorbed into the generally biological. *Hartmann is struggling to confine steadily developing human and personal phenomena within the straitjacket of prepersonal biological concepts.* Psychoanalysis is treated as being about the human organism adapting to the structure of the external world, instead of being about the human psyche realizing its inherent ego-potential for unique individuality as a person relating to other persons. Hartmann is certainly wrong when he says that psychoanalysis is interested in object-relations because they are essential to biological equilibrium. Man's first object-relations are crucial for his biological equilibrium. Without a good mother-infant relationship, the neonate human organism may die, but that is the reason for biology being interested in human object-relations. Psychoanalysis is interested in these relationships for quite different reasons, namely that they are crucial for the achievement of reality and maturity as a person-ego, as Winnicott shows so conclusively.

Hartmann speaks of the environment to which man has to adapt as having two parts, the part not molded by man and the part that has been molded by man; roughly, if not quite accurately, nature and civilization or society. He writes as if in both cases adaptation were the same kind of process, in saying, "The crucial adaptation man has to make is to the social structure, man's adaptation to man." This he calls *social compliance*, coined in analogy to *somatic compliance*, both being special forms of *environmental compliance*. This is the concept of adaptation. Psychoanalysis is then made to rest on the view that the human organism (not person) must adapt by somatic compliance to its natural environment, and by a parallel social compliance to its human environment, these being the twin aspects of environmental compliance as the over-all concept. But at this point Hartmann seems uneasy and writes, "By adaptation we do not mean only passive submission to the goals of society but also active collaboration on them and attempts to change them." [8] This goes beyond biology without admitting it. Attempts to change the environment are not either somatic or social compliance, or adaptation in that sense. If we use concepts strictly, adaptation as compliance can only be autoplastic, altering the organism to fit the environment. Alloplastic change, altering the environment to fit the organism, is not compliance but a highly individual reaction. It is rebellious not adaptive. The animal has little chance of achieving it, having neither the intelligence nor the technology to emulate man. But it is an entirely inadequate concept to represent the intricate processes that go on between the human individual and the social environment, involving mutual understanding and interpersonal relationships.

Thus, when we have accepted man's capacity for alloplastic manipulation of his material environment by scientific technology, and of his human environment by law and power-politics, we have still not arrived at the subject-matter of psychoanalysis. Hartmann, in his theory of environmental compliance, somatic and social, is the purely objective scientist, biological and social, studying human beings from the outside, treating health as a successful adaptation to ensure survival. But physical survival is the business of biology only, not of psychoanalysis. We only reach the level of psychoanalytic concern when either accepting or resisting, complying with or altering the environment, is in the service of quality of personality, not of mere survival of the organism. When a human being challenges or opposes his environment on principle, in defense or pursuit of positive values, seeking to promote more genuine personal relationships, then we are dealing not with biological adaptation to secure survival but with psychodynamic motivation to safeguard the intrinsic quality of personal living. This has often involved not only a Christ or a Socrates but in our time thousands of simple people in the hands of the Gestapo in a refusal to adapt, leading to the destruction of the individual, but the survival of the values for which he died. It is here, with the personal, not the merely organic, that psychoanalysis has its relevance.

Psychoanalysis has to understand the person, the unique individual as he lives and grows in complex meaningful relationships with other persons who are at the same time growing in their relationships with him. This mutual living arises out of biological conditions and goes on in sociological conditions, but it achieves a spiritual independence of both on the level of its own special significance, that of the person-ego in personal relationships. A human being is a psychosomatic whole in which the soma provides the basis of material existence and the machinery for carrying out the purposes of the psychic self. He has bodily appetites and functions to subserve existence, great mental resources, and a latent self that is his *raison d'être* to find and be in the process of relating to his complex material and human environment. This involves that being is more fundamental than doing, quality more fundamental than activity, that the reality of what a man does is determined by what he is, as when a middle-aged woman on a British television program said, "I plunged early into marriage and motherhood, trying to substitute 'doing' for 'being'." In this lies the difference between adapting and relating, which is why I must disagree with Hartmann when he writes, "An investigation such as this one, which uses man's relation to his environment as its point of departure, should focus on action." Adaptation is one-sided and is certainly a matter of action. But personal object-relations are essentially two-sided, mutual by reason of being personal, and not a matter of mutual adaptation merely, but of mutual appreciation, communication, sharing, and of each being for the other.

Hartmann approaches this ultimate problem when he writes, "The question is whether and to what extent, a certain course of development can count on average expectable stimulations (environmental releasers) and whether and to what extent and in what direction it will be deflected by environmental influences of a different kind." He sees that after all the important issue is not the individual adapting to the environment, but the opposite situation, the environment interfering harmfully in the individual's development. The growth of a unique and healthy person is not possible unless the environment can adapt suitably to the needs and potentials of the individual, both supporting and leaving him free for spontaneous growth. It is because, as Hartmann says, "development can be deflected by environmental influences," of a kind not adapted to the individual's needs, that so many people are not able to achieve genuine self-fulfillment and the sense of inner reality as a personal self; and therefore fall into neurosis, crime, suicide, and psychopathology. These are the individual's desperate protests against environments that do not really accept and understand them, and stifle the growth of a true self. Winnicott observes that "good-enough mothering" must be frequent enough, for otherwise the majority of people would display more signs of deep-seated psychosis. On the other hand, when one discovers that quite serious difficulties in conducting the ordinary human relationships are more often the rule than the exception, and that so much of this is hidden behind masks of respectable good behavior, one becomes aware of the subtle "nonacceptances" that great numbers of children suffer at the hands of their respective parents and families. Perhaps the most important thing Fairbairn ever wrote was that the cause of mental illness lay in the fact that "parents fail to get it across to the child that he is loved for his own sake, as a person in his own right." Family and social cultural atmospheres are inextricably mixed in this matter. Thus Erikson describes how Sioux women are culturally subordinated to men. The men are hunters, and the women are simply those who look after the hunters. As a result, suicide is practically unknown among Sioux males, but not infrequent among Sioux females who are only too well adapted to their social environment

and role, which often fails to enable them to achieve genuine
personal selfhood, so that life seems not worth continuing.
The person, the quality of selfhood, is more important than
survival, which is not worthwhile without it.

Winnicott writes of the "average expectable environment"
as essential to the growth of healthy personality in the child,
and the important element in it is "the good-enough mother."
Instead of "courses of development counting on environmental releasers," he writes of *The Maturational Processes and the
Facilitating Environment*. There is a subtle difference. Hartmann's wording conjures up a picture of an innate process
triggered off and pursuing its own autonomous course of development. Winnicott implies a continuously helping, foster-
ing, nursing environment, accepting the infant's immature
dependence while supporting his tentative adventures into independence, individuality, and finding a life of his own in and
through personal relationships.

Winnicott, who was a pediatrician at the Paddington Hospital, London, for forty years, had an unrivaled opportunity
to study mothers and children at all stages, which guided his
adult analyses. Winnicott saw how profoundly the struggles
of the infant and child to grow a real self determine the nature and state of every problem the adult experiences. In *The
Family and Individual Development* he writes of "The First
Year of Life" and "The Relationship of a Mother to her Baby
at the Beginning." His opening words are:

Emotional development starts at the beginning; in a study of the
evolution of the personality and character, it is not possible to
ignore the events of the first days and hours . . . and even birth
experience may be significant. The world has kept turning in spite
of our ignorance in these matters, simply because there is something about the mother of a baby, something which makes her
particularly suited to the protection of her infant in this stage
of vulnerability and which makes her able to contribute positively to the baby's positive needs. The mother is able to fulfil

this role if she feels secure; if she feels loved in her relation to the infant's father and to her family; and also accepted in the widening circles around the family which constitute society. . . . Her capacity does not rest on knowledge but comes from a feeling attitude which she acquires as pregnancy advances, and which she gradually loses as the infant grows up out of her.[9]

I regard this factual statement, as the fruit of years of first-hand experience, as completely nullifying speculative theories of a death instinct, and of aggression as an innate primary destructive drive. If human infants are not surrounded by genuine love from birth, radiating outward into a truly caring family and social environment, then we pay for our failure toward the next generation by having to live in a world torn with fear and hate, full of grossly unhappy people who wreck marriages and friendships and constantly swell the ranks of the deeply disturbed, from unproductive hippies living in a flimsy fantasy world, to criminals, delinquents, and psychopaths. In between are the all too common fanatical adherents of scientific, political, economic, educational, and religious ideologies trying to call or drive us to various types of earthly paradise, and always failing to devote their resources to the one necessary thing, achieving a recognition of the fact that the importance of security for babies and mother outweighs every other issue. If that is not achieved, everything else we do merely sustains human masses to struggle on from crisis to crisis, from minor to major breakdowns. Today the world may not "keep turning in spite of our ignorance in these matters" much longer. Nor do we want hordes of would-be scientific educators teaching psychology to mothers, for the mother's ability to give her baby a secure start in life "does not depend on knowledge but on a feeling" that comes naturally if she herself feels secure. Winnicott writes, "It is often possible to detect and diagnose emotional disorder in . . . the first year of life. The right time for the treatment of such disorder is the time of its inception." [10] This is the overriding fact that should determine our social goals. It is therefore essential to construct psychoanalytic theory on the right factual basis and in the right intellectual atmosphere, which is not that of objective material science. If that had always been appreciated, psychodynamic theories would have been spared many absurdities.

The capacity of the secure mother to provide security for her baby is described by Winnicott as "primary maternal preoccupation." He writes:

We notice in the expectant mother an increasing identification with the infant . . . and a willingness as well as an ability on the part of the mother to drain interest from her own self onto the baby . . . This is the thing that gives the mother her special ability to do the right thing. She knows what the baby could be feeling like. No one else knows. Doctors and nurses may know a lot about psychology and of course they know all about body health and disease. But they do not know what a baby feels like from minute to minute because they are outside this area of experience.[11]

He observes that the disturbed, compulsive, or pathologically preoccupied mother "fails to plunge into this extraordinary experience which is almost like an illness, though it is very much a sign of mental health." Finally, "It is part of the normal process that the mother recovers her self-interest, and does so at the rate at which her infant can allow her to do so."[12] Thus, the mother gives the infant a start in life, in a condition of as near perfect security as we can imagine, in a human relationship that involves total physical and emotional dependence, and then gradually lets him grow an increasing measure of independence of her, so that he can become a separate individual without disturbing the now permanent, built-in sense of belonging, relationship, and security at heart. In this ideal start, dependence and independence do not become conflicting issues, rather they are complementary. In the first discussion I ever had with Fairbairn, he said, "Dependence versus independence is the basic neurotic conflict. The person one turns to becomes the person one must get away from." I did not then realize the depth and ramifications of that statement. It describes the schizoid "in and out" conflict. Its origin lies in the failure of initial mothering to provide both support and freedom, to foster both relationship and individuality.

Winnicott carries us a stage further with his important concept of "basic ego-relatedness." This conceptualizes what a good-enough mother-infant relationship does for the child, in terms of built-in experience that will last for a lifetime as a foundation on which all the child's later growth can take place. In a paper on "The Capacity to Be Alone," a capacity that is "one of the most important signs of maturity in emotional development," he links this with basic ego-relatedness. Thus toward the end of a successful treatment, a silent session may indicate the patient's maturity and self-possession. He no longer needs to talk to feel sure of his relationship with the therapist. The mature person can enjoy solitude and privacy without feeling any loss of relationship; indeed it may be essential to creativity. This "sophisticated aloneness" is built on "a capacity to be alone . . . which is a phenomenon of early life." [13] Winnicott writes:

Although many types of experience go to the establishment of the capacity to be alone, there is one that is basic; without a sufficiency of it the capacity to be alone does not come about; *this experience is that of being alone, as an infant and small child, in the presence of mother.* Thus the basis of the capacity to be alone is a paradox; it is the experience of being alone while someone else is present. Here is implied a rather special type of relationship, that between the infant or small child who is alone, and the mother who is, in fact, reliably present even if represented for the moment by a cot or a pram or the general atmosphere of the immediate environment. . . . For this special type of relationship, I like to use the term *ego-relatedness* . . . Ego-relatedness refers to the relationship between two people, one of whom at any rate is alone; perhaps both are alone, yet the presence of each is important to the other.[14]

Finally Winnicott describes ego-relatedness as the sharing of "a solitude that is relatively free from the property that we call 'withdrawal'."

What he is here describing is the way in which an infant who starts life in a state of total emotional identification with his mother can begin to experience his separateness from her, without losing the experience of relatedness, provided his "ego-immaturity is naturally balanced by ego-support from the mother." The sense of belonging, of being securely in touch that grows in the baby from the mother's loving reliability, becomes an established property of his psyche. He does not feel he has lost his mother when he cannot see her, he does not feel isolated when he is physically alone. The subtle transitional stage between feeling securely related when mother is holding him, and still feeling securely related when mother is absent, is, Winnicott suggests, a stage in which the baby who is actually with his mother can forget about her while she is still there because he feels nothing but security toward her. The baby gains proof that his trust is justified by remembering his mother again and finding that she is still there. Then in time he can tolerate her actual absence with no feeling of having lost her or of being alone in the world. Winnicott elaborates this with a useful formula. The baby comes to be able to bear the mother's absence for x minutes, but she must then come back to him to prevent his mental image of her from fading for then he would feel as if he had lost her. If she is away $x + y$ minutes, all may not be lost if she can restore his fading image of her by special mothering and spoiling. But if she is away $x + y + z$ minutes, then when she returns to the baby she is a stranger to him, and his ego has begun to disintegrate. He has, as it were, fallen into a

mental vacuum of ego-unrelatedness. That is the essential definition of the schizoid state. When patients develop acute
anxiety states with feelings of isolation, unreality, and nonentity, they are reexperiencing that basic ego-unrelatedness
caused by maternal failure in infancy. Many people hover between feeling not quite lost and out of touch but not con-
vincingly in touch. A reviewer of a biography of T. H.
White, the author, said, "His troubled heart was an inner
emptiness, a failure to achieve human attachment." "Human
attachment" has to be given to us as infants, if we are to be
able to become secure as adults. Moreover, those who do not
have this experience as part of their basic personality make-up
are excessively vulnerable even to the slightest risk of loss of
support. Their chronic over-dependency is a genuine compulsion that they cannot, by effort or will-power, not feel.
Their only hope is to find someone who can understand this
and help them to grow out of it. This is what psychotherapy
is. The innermost schizoid core of a depersonalized human
being is very difficult to reach for complex reasons. It is (1)
withdrawn and regressed in fear, (2) repressed because the
weak infant is unacceptable to consciousness, (3) disintegrated in the beginnings of its ego-structure, thus feeling unreal and not a proper person, and (4) most profoundly of all,
unevoked in its potentialities, never fully called to life in the
unfacilitating environment.

Thus, we arrive at the radical theory of the object-relational
origins of the person-ego. Apart from interpersonal relations,
an ego or true self never develops at all, and as Spitz made
clear, the too gravely unmothered infant may even die. In
"The Location of Cultural Experience," Winnicott hints at
the far-reaching implications of the facts that this theory
conceptualizes. He takes up his earlier concept of the transitional object, the soft toy or article that the infant will not
part with, in the period when he is beginning to realize that
he and his mother are separate objects, and that she can be

out of sight. The toy that mother has given him comes to his rescue if he becomes anxious. It reminds him of her, stands for her and her reliability, and keeps alive his mental image of her until she comes back in time to reassure him personally. She makes his experience of her feel reliable and makes his transitional object a reliable representation of her reality. Winnicott suggests that this toy is the very first definite symbol of relationship, and is actually the beginning of culture. Culture is the ever-expanding elaboration of our symbols for representing our life as persons, as consisting in the meaningful development of our personalities toward maturity in those interpersonal relations that are the very stuff of living. The whole of art, literature, and religion are embraced in culture in this sense. Science is not a part of culture, being a more pedestrian, utilitarian thing, however much its studies of our expanding universe stimulate our imagination. If ego-unrelatedness is the essence of the schizoid state of depersonalization, unreality, and nonentity, then ego-relatedness is the foundation of the experience of ego-reality and selfhood, the feeling of inbeingness as a definite self.

The problem of having an unquestioned possession or else a lack of a sense of personal reality and selfhood, the identity problem, is the biggest single issue that can be raised about human existence. It has always been the secret critical issue; only in our time have we become explicitly conscious of it. In an as yet unpublished paper on "The Female and Male Elements in Human Bisexuality," Winnicott regards the female element as being and the male element as doing, both factors existing in both males and females, if with somewhat different emphases. Against this standard we can assess the neurotic distortions of masculinity and femininity encountered not only in patients but in popular opinion; the identification of female with weak, making some women despise their own sex and produce Adler's "masculine protest"; and of "male" with strength, which then usually means aggressiveness.

Freud's most unfortunate mistake was to regard aggression, destructiveness, as in itself a primary instinctive drive, a death instinct. The more primitive the society, the more aggression becomes simply self-defense. Margaret Mead described a peaceful tribe in which there is a minimum of distinction between the sexes, where boys and girls played cooperative and gentle games together, and both parents were equally interested in the raising of children, giving them plenty of love and attention. The more complex societies become, the more fears and insecurities create vicious circles of suspicion, defensiveness, defense by attack, and counterattack. An aggressive society becomes self-perpetuating, a nearly insoluble problem. But we must not blindly ascribe this to nature and instinct. It is a sign of the bankruptcy of the creative capacities to live and love. Being, the sense of assured stable selfhood, is the basis of healthy doing, of spontaneous creative activity. Without it, doing can only be forced self-driving to keep oneself going, a state of mind that breeds aggression, in the first place against oneself; and then to gain some relief from self-persecution, it is turned outward against other people, situations, or causes, creating the social neuroses of fanaticism, political, religious, or idiosyncratic.

Finally, Winnicott distinguishes between orgiastic and non-orgiastic experiences; that is, between the experience of the satisfaction of instinct, which waxes and wanes, and has to do with Freud's concepts of tension-relieving gratification; and the quite different experience of personal relating, which is far more profound, persisting, and the permanent basis of reliable ego-experience. Instinct-satisfaction has little to do with this. A baby's hunger can be satisfied, but it still needs to stay at the breast, not for food but for relationship. Fairbairn told me of a patient who said that his baby was always crying and losing weight, so Fairbairn advised a change of food, as the baby was not being breast fed. The result was that the baby gained weight and was soon back to a normal weight, but was crying as much as ever, so Fairbairn arranged for an experienced social worker to visit the home. She reported that the mother was propping the bottle on a cushion and merely watching to see that the baby got the food, but was not nursing it. She explained to this young mother the importance of nursing for the baby's emotional needs. Fairbairn's patient later reported that the baby hardly ever cried now and was doing well. If the mother leaves the baby alone too long, it becomes emotionally traumatized. In Winnicott's words:

The baby has experienced unthinkable anxiety . . . the acute confusional state that belongs to disintegration of whatever ego-structure existed at the time. . . . Emotional growth ceases. . . . Madness is the breakup of whatever may exist at the time of a personal existence. . . . A baby has to start again permanently deprived of its own root, which would be a continuity with the personal beginning.[15]

If the mother does not allow this tragedy to happen, then the baby develops a "capacity to use a symbol of union: the baby then comes to allow and benefit from separation."

Winnicott specifically distinguished "this field of the bodily relationship between baby and mother" from the quite different "oral erotism with satisfaction." He says:

The phenomena I am describing (that is, basic secure personal relations) have no climax. This distinguishes them from phenomena that have instinctual backing, where the orgiastic element plays an essential part and where satisfactions are closely linked with climax. . . . Psychoanalysts who have rightly emphasized the significance of instinctual experience and reaction to frustration have failed to state with comparable clearness or conviction the tremendous intensity of these nonclimactic experiences of relating to objects.[16]

Psychoanalytic theory dealing with conflicts over, and defenses against, instincts, has, he states:

not yet started to describe life apart from illness, i.e. to tackle the question of what life is about. . . . We now see that it is not instinctual satisfaction that makes a baby begin to be, to feel that life is real, to find life worth living. . . . The self must precede the self's use of instinct. The rider must ride the horse, not be run away with it.[17]

He clinches this by commenting, "I can see that I am in the territory of Fairbairn's (1941) concept of object-seeking (as opposed to satisfaction-seeking)." [18]

It is revolutionary, from the classic psychoanalytic point of view to subordinate instinct phenomena as partial experiences, to the living whole of the person-ego growing in and only as a result of good enough personal relations experience. In the longer version of the 1967 paper as originally read, Winnicott asked:

Should I pause to discover whether I have company or am alone? Are there those who think that the most intense experiences belong to instinctual and orgiastic events? I do wish to make it quite clear that I believe this would be wrong and dangerously wrong. The statement leaves out of account the function of the ego-organization. Only if someone is there adding up personal experience into a total that can become a self does instinctual satisfaction avoid becoming a disrupting factor, or have a meaning beyond its localized meaning as a sample of physiology. . . . What is life about? You may cure your patient and not know what it is that makes him or her go on living. The first step is to acknowledge openly that absence of psychoneurotic illness may be health but it is not life. Psychotic patients who are all the time hovering between living and not living force us to look at this problem, which really belongs not to psychoneurosis but to all human beings. I am claiming that these same phenomena which are life and death to our schizoid patients essentially appear in our cultural experience.[19]

All in all I think that this is the most revolutionary bit of writing yet produced within psychoanalysis. Its insight could not have been reached without all of the preliminary investigations into neurosis, sex, aggression, guilt, ego-splitting, and the internal-objects world, but it is the true goal of all that Freud started, that is, an understanding of how we become persons in personal relationships, of how mankind has sought to express the significance of this personal living in the growing body of culture through the ages. The most far-reaching questions were raised when Winnicott asked: "What is life about? You may cure your patient and not know what it is that makes him or her go on living. . . . Absence of psychoneurotic illness may be health but it is not life." He certainly only used the term "cure" *en passant*. It is not a term psychoanalysts often use, and one of which even physicians are chary. The most obvious meaning that can be given to it is abolition of symptoms. For the behavior therapist this is cure, for the psychoanalyst it certainly is not. Often the existence and continuance of symptoms is what motivates the patient to seek therapy, the real aim of which is to open the way for radical changes in personality, in areas relevant to the production of the symptoms. Symptoms indicate the real nature of the trouble, and that which deals not with illness (i.e., symptoms of disturbed functioning) but with whether or not this patient feels real as a person. If he does not, he will be subject to anxieties of every sort and incapable, according to the degree of his basic unreality as a person, of living any satisfactory life either for himself or in relation to other people. Ultimately, these mental illnesses are not strictly speaking medical matters at all. The control of symptoms when they are too crippling and indicate severe basic personality failure is a medical matter, and often psychoanalytic therapy cannot be carried on without such medical aid. In the end, however, the solution is not in the realm of medicine as professionally understood. It is in the realm of personal relationships, of the growth of personal reality within oneself, of life having a worthwhile meaning (because it can and does become significant only when, and in so far as, genuine personal relationships can be made). No wonder Freud held that a medical training was not enough for, and might even be in many respects irrelevant to, the training of a psychoanalyst. Though he did not provide the psychological basis for an understanding of culture, he did include a knowledge of culture (literature, art, and religion) as necessary for psycho-analytic therapy, since such therapy is in the end concerned with "what life is about" rather than with simply health. It is in the line of the logical development of psychoanalysis that Winnicott has raised this question and given us a basis for a psychology of culture; for culture is man's continuing struggle to define and express what his life means to him.

To summarize, a human infant can only grow to be a person-ego, a self, out of his original state of total mergence in and identification with his mother prior to birth, if the mother's ego support for him after birth is adequate through the period of his separating out from her mentally. Then, as a strongly formed personal self with an unshakable deep experience of basic ego-relatedness as a built-in foundation for future growth, the adult socialized ego develops the mature capacity both to be alone without feeling isolated, and to commit and involve himself in true self-devotion, or even apparent self-abnegation for adequate reasons, without losing his proper individuality. This perhaps is the peak of maturity (unfortunately easily neurotically counterfeited), to be able to give oneself to the utmost in love, for convincing reasons, without loss of ego-integrity. The model for this is the mature mother with her baby, which, as Winnicott says, may look like illness but is in fact the supreme mark of health; that is, not infatuation but genuine self-giving. This must also be the mature way of falling in love, which need not therefore be, as Freud seems to have thought, a neurotic infatuation. It must also be the hallmark of mature friendship of every degree, and finally of the psychotherapeutic relationship. Perhaps it is the reality of genuine religious experiences, which needs exploration.

A comparison of the work of Edith Jacobson with that of Hartmann and Winnicott will further clarify this position. As with an increasing number of workers in this field, Jacobson's attention has been forced to concentrate on the problems of the formation of the ego and the development of ego-identity, by

the widening scope of psychoanalysis and the growing number of borderline or even psychotic patients who call on the analyst for help. In such patients we can observe processes of regression that lead to a grave deterioration of object-relations and of super-ego and ego functions, with dissolution of those essential identifications on which the experience of our personal identity is founded.[20]

At once this raises the critical question of whether the persistence of these "essential identifications" is really that on which "the experience of our personal identity is founded." May they not have more to do with that basic ego-weakness that later emerges as breakdown into borderline or psychotic illness, when regression to the earliest underlying psychic states occurs. Freud regarded identifications as substitutes for lost or broken-down object-relationships. If Winnicott is right, the basis of ego-strength is created in the object-relationship of the baby to the mother as the infant emerges from its primary identification or psychophysical oneness with her. Thereafter, identifications with parents and other people play important roles in furthering the development of the whole personality, but transiently and at different stages. The persistence of early identifications must create a false identity, which is not a natural development of the child's own individuality. This leads to ego-rigidity, and unless early identifications are dissolved and replaced by real object-relations that promote natural self-development, a true self-identity cannot be found. This does not imply that perfection is attainable in this matter, but that the degree of health and maturity depends on this process.

This plunges us deeply into Jacobson's views of the nature of the primary symbiotic mother-infant relationship, and of the process by which the differentiation of subject and object, mother and infant proceeds. She concludes that Freud's formulations in "The Ego and The Id" concerning the starting point are "rather ambiguous . . . quite puzzling and require elucidation." [21] His view in *The Outline of Psychoanalysis* of "an initial state of things in the as yet undifferentiated ego-id" in which "libido . . . serves to neutralize the destructive impulses which are simultaneously present" [22] poses insuperable problems for his concepts of primary narcissism and primary masochism. They cannot have any significance "in the primary psychic organization prior to the child's discovery of his own self and the object-world." [23] This is a point Melanie Klein failed to see, in adopting the mystical Eros and Thanatos theory. Thus Jacobson feels "compelled to dispose of the concept of primary masochism, that is, of Freud's death instinct theory . . . (as) rather speculative." [24] She writes:

We may wonder whether the observable facts might not be explained more readily by the assumption that, at the very beginning of life, the instinctual energy is still in an undifferentiated state: and that from birth on it develops into two kinds of psychic drives with different qualities under the influence of external situations, of psychic growth and the opening up of increasing maturation of pathways for outside discharge. [25]

Thus libidinal and aggressive drives are no longer innate as separate entities to become secondary manifestations in the postnatal infant. They are seen by Jacobson as "setting in at the stage of beginning ego-formation" and of the distinguishing of objects from each other and from the self, and "their different representations in the now system-ego gradually become endowed with an enduring libidinal and aggressive cathexis." [26]

I find myself in close agreement with this except for the

fact that the use of the term "system-ego" is a warning of problems to be faced. Jacobson appears to be unacquainted in the 1950s with Fairbairn's work of the early 1940s but thus far their positions are closely related. In Fairbairn's terms there is a pristine whole psychosomatic self, however primitive, at the start. Jacobson, too, rejected the death instinct and saw the development of libidinal and aggressive drives after birth as a result of object-relations experience. Jacobson tries to retain some value for the concept of primary narcissism as "a useful term for the earliest infantile period, preceding the development of self and object images, the stage during which the infant is as yet unaware of anything but his own experiences of tension and relief, of frustration and gratification."[27] Any argument for retaining primary narcissism would apply equally well to primary masochism, and we must retain or reject both. Moreover, narcissism is far too sophisticated a term (Narcissus falling in love with his own image in its reflection in a pool) to be relevant as a description of what Jacobson calls "the primary undifferentiated psychosomatic matrix" and the "primal psychophysiological self," or to the infant's subjective state *in utero* and in the earliest infantile postnatal sleep that Freud regarded as "reproducing intrauterine existence."[28] Jacobson writes: "The depressed or catatonic stuporous states appear to be pathological versions of the infant's dozing states," but she points out that "these pathological regressed states . . . show convincing evidence of destructive or self-destructive processes . . . of which we find no signs in the normal state of sleep, and in the early infantile childhood state. Quite the contrary . . . the sleeping state has a recuperative function."[29] It is pertinent to remark that if there were libidinal and destructive impulses simultaneously present in the infant *in utero,* as Freud and Melanie Klein held, then sleep could not have a truly recuperative function. Sleep is not primary narcissism but detachment from the consciously experienced outer-world, while much mental activity concerned with ego development goes on in a state of near conscious self-awareness, while in a condition of over-all unselfconscious relaxed security. In the insecure ego sleep is disturbed. There can be no narcissism prior to ego-development, and then only an insecure ego has motives for developing marked narcissistic self-concern, as distinct from the natural energetic self-assertive activity of the growing child, which is part of the process of ego-development and consolidation.

Jacobson proposes a true object-relational theory of ego-develópment. Primary narcissism and masochism, the differentiation of libido and aggression prior to any object-relations experience, prior to birth, are replaced by the necessities, difficulties, anxieties, needs, and insecurities experienced in the early growth of the undifferentiated psyche-soma with its potential for becoming a viable ego, as separation of subject and object takes place. In this process libidinal and aggressive drives develop: not as drives that were there before the differentiation of subject and object, but drives that are developing ego-reactions to real good and bad external objects. The development of the ego, and of drives differentiated appropriately to the nature of the object-world, and the development of increasingly definite perception of objects and their nature, all proceed together. Gradually, the beginnings of ego structure are consolidated on the basis of primary ego-relatedness, if that experience has become built-in by a good mother-infant relationship. Libido is the essential life-energy, the urge to object-relations, the drive of the growing ego or self to live by relating to its environment.

At this point, however, it becomes clear that Jacobson has not fully freed herself of the idea so common in psycho-analysis, and necessitated by instinct-theory, that aggression must somehow be original, an inborn factor in its own right. Her acceptance of Freud's dual theory of drives, libidinal and aggressive, still places both of them on the same footing. This is apparent in the attempt she makes, but cannot carry through successfully, to use the distinction between "drives inwards" and "drives outwards." Jacobson admits:

during infancy and even in early childhood it is not easy to discern the aggressive and libidinal qualities of the child's instinctual and emotional manifestations, and that such affective phenomena as anxiety and rage still appear to be closely interwoven. While such a conception may be reminiscent of the frustration-aggression theory, it should be noted that the transformation of the undifferentiated psychophysiological energy into two qualitatively different kinds of psychic drives is here regarded as psychobiologically predetermined, and as promoted by internal maturational as well as external stimuli.[30]

This allows observation to be overridden by theory, and confuses two different issues. The observation recorded is that it is not easy to discern distinct libidinal and aggressive qualities, and that rage shows as a reaction to anxiety. That is the observation that gave rise to the frustration-aggression theory. Carrying the observation further, from infancy to psychotherapy, in twenty-five years of psychoanalytic therapy I have not come across any case of unanalyzable aggression, that is, I have always found that all forms of aggressive reaction were defensive reactions to fears, anxieties, insecurities, feelings of underlying weakness, and especially basic feelings of isolation. Ernest Jones, in a deeply interesting paper, "The Concept of a Normal Mind" has highly pertinent things to say about this.

It is certain that much of what passes as "strength of character" is an illusion. Such traits as obstinacy, pugnacity . . . hardness of heart, insensitiveness to the feelings of other human beings, however useful they may on occasion be to their owner, are often little more than defenses against love of which the person is too afraid. . . . A matter-of-fact attitude of being "superior to sentiment" is often a buttressing of the personality, a self-justification in the presence of deep seated fear.[31]

Observing that the capacity for friendliness and affection depends on "internal freedom," he continues,

Inner confidence and security enable the person to endure opposition calmly and to be so unintimidated by hostility as to render aggressive opposition on his part unnecessary except in extreme and urgent situations.[32]

He calls this characteristic of maturity "confident sereneness," and it clearly depends on the absence of fear, the presence of self-confidence, and the lack of need to react aggressively. My own conviction that fear is always the root cause of aggression, which cannot therefore be a "psychological *ultimate*" factor *per se*, is reinforced by Jones's further elaborations on this theme. He writes:

Personally I have long shared the opinion, expressed more than half a century ago by a German writer, Dick (1877), that anxiety is the Alpha and Omega of psychiatry. I would unhesitatingly extend this view to the field of normal psychology, and maintain that on the way in which any individual deals with *the primordial anxiety of infancy* more depends than on anything else in development. Fear is the most fundamental member of the triad of fear, hate, and guilt.[33]

Finally:

We reach the conclusion that the nearest attainable criterion of normality is fearlessness. The most normal person is, like Siegfried, *angstfrei*, but we must be clear that we mean by this not merely manifest courage, but the absence of all the deep reactions that mask unconscious apprehensiveness. Where these are absent we have the willing or even joyful acceptance of life, with all its visitations and chances, that distinguishes the free personality of one who is master of himself.[34]

In spite of Jones's acceptance of Freud's theory of aggression as biological instinct (although Jones himself rejected the death instinct theory), the inference that must be drawn from

Jones's clinical observations is that aggression is a secondary manifestation that occurs only as a direct result of, and re-action to, fear. Jacobson, having made the same observations of the infant, unnecessarily qualifies it by viewing aggression as one of two "qualitatively different kinds of psychic drives, here regarded as psychobiologically predetermined."

In fact, what Jacobson does here is what so many writers have done with this problem of aggression. It is confused and equated with natural assertiveness, the energetic life-drive that in its basic nature is not aggressive but vitally libidinal. As Fairbairn stated, "The goal of libido is the object," and if the object is good, the normal reaction is love. It is this active, assertive, libidinal drive that is "psychobiologically predeter-mined" and "promoted by internal maturational as well as ex-ternal stimuli." It is when frustration or threat are met with and fear is aroused that the infant must either flee or fight, and since he cannot physically do either, the result of the far too early arousal of fear is the gross undermining of the ego. Aggression in later life is most usually caused by a desperate struggle to overcome this basic weakness. Of course, overt aggressive reactions are not possible until "maturational processes" consolidate at least some amount of ego-structure and place at its disposal increasingly developed muscular and sensory powers. This, however, does not imply that these "maturational processes" develop the aggressive drive per se. That is always a reaction to a bad-object world. The frus-tration-aggression theory is the only one supported by clinical observation, and is really implied in Jacobson's object-relational theory of the origin of drives and ego-growth as starting together after birth. With the discarding of any dif-ferentiation between primary and secondary narcissism and masochism, and the rejection of the so-called primary drives, we are free to base our concepts strictly on clinical evidence and not on speculation. Narcissism and masochism can be analyzed as they are seen in patients' dreams and symptoms, as pathological ego-states expressing internalized good and bad object-relations (in Melanie Klein's sense). These arise out of the loss of external real-life object-relations and their replacement by identifications with internalized objects. Freud described this process in mourning and depression as the installing of the lost loved and hated object in the ego.

Here is a clinically verifiable use of the concepts of "drives to the inside" and "drives to the outside," in object-relational terms. Jacobson, however, although she has emancipated herself from the classical psychoanalytic theory, cannot escape its influence or fully disown it, and brings it back again by seeking once more to base these psychodynamic concepts on pure biology, falling back on "drives to the inside" and the necessity for "neutralized energy" concepts. She writes, "Psychic life originates in physiological processes which are independent of external sensory stimulations. From birth on, however, the discharge processes expand with the opening up of biologically predetermined and preferred pathways for discharge in response to external stimulation." [35] Also "In contradistinction to the 'silent' predominantly psychophysiological discharge of the embryo or newborn or during sleep, the emotions of the adult find expression not only in secretory, circulatory, respiratory phenomena indicative of physiological discharge towards the inside, but also in patterned motor phenomena and in the inner perceptions which we call feelings, *i.e.*, in manifestation of discharge towards the outside." [36] However, we cannot say that "Psychic life *originates* in physiological processes," which are purely internal, and independent of external sensory stimuli. The fertilized cell is the product of two adult psychosomatic whole persons, and both aspects, psycho and somatic must develop together from the start. This becomes distinguishable (for our thinking) in the first discernible movements of the unborn embryo inside the womb. In some dim way the inside of the uterus at that stage must have become the first "environment" of the unborn baby, and object-relations experience has already found its vaguest origins before the traumatic experience of birth. We also know now that the unborn baby reacts to light and noise. Thus must the differentiation of subject and object have its first barely perceptible beginnings early, and birth must provide the first large-scale stimulus for its clearer development, the rate of which depends on the maturation of brain and sensory organs. Prior to birth, activity must be conceived as neither libidinal nor aggressive in any sense in which these are opposed, but just vital and energetic. If Freud is right that anxiety begins with the birth-trauma, then that also is the first clear situation in which fear must begin the generation of incipient aggression, which can be speedily allayed by what Winnicott calls good-enough mothering. From then on, the differentiation of specific libidinal and aggressive drives will depend on the object-relations experience of the baby. Jacobson's need to distinguish between drives to the inside and drives to the outside is really determined by her need to believe that aggression as well as libido is biologically predetermined, and therefore innate after all. The truth appears to me to be that there is one basic psychophysiological life-drive toward the object-world, which generates fear and aggression when thwarted.

This theory eliminates the purely speculative and clinically impossible idea of neutralized energy made available for the use of the ego and superego. This idea presupposes the id-ego theory, which would only really be viable if it could be proved that there are id-drives, both libidinal and aggressive, before birth and that the ego only begins to be after birth. Once we substitute for this speculative idea the concept of a psychosomatic whole with ego-potential, developing primarily libidinally in object-relations, but also aggressively if thwarted, then the ego is the whole psychic person, the psychic aspect of the basic psychosomatic whole being. This person-ego has its own energy or life-drive, and develops a structural identity and individual characteristics by organizing its experiences as it goes along. There is no place for the idea of neutralizing original sexual and aggressive id-drives to make a pale characterless energy, neutralized and available to a system-ego that has no proper energy of its own. This concept belongs only in the context of Hartmann's system-ego theory and its inherent self-contradiction was recognized even by Rapaport and Erikson. Thus Apfelbaum writes of Hartmann, "ego, as intellect and judgement, freed from emotion as represented by the id, based on neutralization and autonomy," and adds, "Erikson questions this view . . . and argues that mechanization and independence of emotion characterize the impoverished ego rather than the healthy one." "Likewise Rapaport observes that the most autonomous ego is the obsessional one. . . . To avoid this danger of overvaluing inhibition and control, the ego psychologists suggest that the efficient ego is capable of giving up its autonomy and reversing the process of neutralization," in order to recover "by regression in the service of the ego, gratifying sexual functioning, the capacity for untroubled sleep, and successful creative activity." [37] One can only ask why neutralization had to be undertaken at all if it must be surrendered in order to possess a healthy ego. This entire speculative concept is clearly unreal.

In everyday usage, the term "aggression" is, indissolubly bound up with the ideas of fighting, hostility, and destructiveness, and in classical Freudian theory it is equated with sadism, destructiveness, and the death instinct. When in everyday parlance we speak of a person as being aggressive, we do not mean that he is healthily and energetically alive and courageous in grappling with practical difficulties. We mean that he is "a nasty piece of work," offensively critical, quarrelsome, bad tempered, and given to trying to get his own way by intimidating others. This is not a manifestation of natural instinct. Anthony Storr, in *Human Aggression* writes:

It is the failure to distinguish between aggression and hatred which has led naive liberal humanists to label all aggression as "bad," and which has led them to hold the ridiculous belief that if human beings were never frustrated, they would not be aggressive at all.[38]

Though I am generally in fairly close agreement with what Storr writes, I am constrained to disagree with him here. Storr regards aggression as a biological necessity, but this I believe involves exactly the same semantic confusion that we have already noted. Is it not the failure to recognize that in actual usage "aggression" *means* "hatred," and the failure is to distinguish between "aggression-hatred" on the one hand, and the vitality, energy, courage, and persistence on the other, with which the healthy minded person grapples against the real difficulties nature plants across our path to biological survival, and other people oppose to our need for personal ego-growth? The African Bushmen showed indomitable courage when, left to themselves, they not only survived but developed a culture and an art in mastering the appalling conditions of existence in the Kalahari Desert. Yet they remained a peaceable and friendly people. They encountered aggression only when they were invaded by already culturally disturbed black marauders from the north and white marauders from the south. Ernest Jones, in tracing aggression to deep-seated fears stored in the unconscious from infancy, and in tracing the absence of aggression to the existence of basic ego-strength, forcibly supports Winnicott's theory of basic-ego-relatedness, the product of really good mother-infant relations, as the foundation of both mental health and personality-maturity.

Healthy competitiveness in sports has nothing in common with aggression as it is fostered in all of us today by the vicious circles of fears, defenses, counterdefenses, more fears that attack is the best form of defense, political stability only being precariously maintained by a balance of terror. All this atmosphere of aggression is based on fear, fed by distinctions between the wealthy and the backward nations, and the rich and the poor in affluent societies, and the unremitting propaganda of violence and aggression poured forth by television, radio, paperback books of the James Bond variety, and pornographic sadism. While scanning a main London railway station bookstall recently, with its paperback racks displaying, with monotonous regularity, cover pictures of revolvers, naked women, men and women lying on the ground wounded, their faces expressing every possible variety of the contorted features of vicious hate, my eye lighted on *The War Babies* by Gwen Davis, a Corgi Book. In the center of the cover I read the following:

"It's got everything. Violence, Sex, Pathos, Sex, Humour, Sex, Racial angles, Sex, the Devastating Effect of War, Sex, Abnormal Psychology, Sex." This was a quotation, presumably from a review from *The Detroit Free Press*. Is it just fussiness to direct straight criticism against this stream of high-powered suggestion of neurotic sexuality and violence?

An American experiment should be considered here. A group of small children was shown a television film of a group of small children attacking another child. They were then taken into another room in the center of which was a life-size doll-child, and they all immediately rushed at it and began to pummel and kick it. People are being culturally conditioned today to accept the combination of sexuality and violence as natural in a way that was never possible before the invention of the modern mass media of communication. Cyril Connolly, reviewing Storr's *Human Aggression*, wrote: "Competition will always trigger off aggressiveness, and society cannot exist without it." As a reaction of "an ordinary common sense person," I quote a letter from *The Yorkshire Post*. The writer refers to events that took place in English County Cricket, and attempts made to condone the attitude that "in going all out to win, the determination to succeed justifies whatever methods are adopted." His pertinent comment was:

What a joy to witness on the Centre Court at Wimbledon, a player in the person of Judy Tegart who was obviously keen on success at international level, but who played the game throughout most generously, and wound up with a display of good sportsmanship in favour of her successful opponent. The suggestion that games at high competitive level cannot be played all out without some degree of friction and unpleasantness was completely negatived by this charming girl from Australia.[39]

I have deliberately chosen here to introduce a point of view from an ordinary nonspecialist source, because it seems to me that so-called scientific thought on this matter could use an injection of plain common-sense.

It is difficult to see how Freud, in starting to explore a hitherto unexplored field, that of human nature in the psychological depths, could have done otherwise as early as the 1890s than make use of the existing concept of "instinct." Nevertheless, there is reason to believe that his theories of instinctive sex and instinctive aggression have done as much harm to our general cultural orientation in this century, especially in the atmospheres engendered by two world wars, as his opening up of the field of psychotherapy in depth has done good. Instead of seeking explanations of aggression in biology, we would do better to concentrate on studying the manifold ways in which the methods of rearing children by parents who themselves had to grow up in aggression-saturated societies disturb the majority of human beings from the start. The present-day importation of so much naked aggression into sport itself, which is alien to its true nature, comes not from enjoyable recreational competition, but from the commercialization of sport, which has its roots in all the fears that breed the money is power complex. If liberal humanists are naive, as they may well be, it is because they do not face the enormously complicated ways in which fear, aggression, counter-aggression, and more fear for centuries has been woven into the minutest details of all social organization. Yet when the intrepid sailors of the Kon Tiki raft, drifting across the Pacific Ocean, ran ashore on an isolated Pacific island, they found a simple and naturally happy and friendly native population, untouched and unspoiled by all that we call civilization. I do not deny for a moment that, as a matter of fact, all human infants do, probably from the start, develop feelings and fantasies of destructive aggression, but that does not prove that aggression is a biologically innate destructive instinct per se, but only that frustration and fear are encountered, according to Freud, from the very beginning in the birth-trauma. That this early anxiety can be allayed by good mothering is beyond dispute. That in the majority of cases this does not happen often because mothers, nurses, and doctors do not understand the emotional implications for personality-formation, is just as obvious. If "aggression" were used in its strictly etymological sense as derived from the Latin *ad* and *gradior* meaning "to step toward," it could well be used for our innate and biologically based will to live and energetic striving to relate to our environment, but it is not thus used. Even the *Oxford Dictionary* defined "aggression" as "beginning a quarrel, unprovoked attack," and *The Students English Dictionary* defines it as "to commit the first act of violence." It is under conditions of fear and real or imagined threat to the ego or total self that this occurs. That the well informed have begun to understand that this kind of fear is rooted in the unconscious of infancy is shown by the review of Storr's book by Cyril Connolly, where he writes: "Infants at the breast are seething with anger . . . Children enter adult life with the subconscious memory of real or fancied injustice to trigger off their aggressiveness into hate. It would be truer to say, 'To adulterate their healthy and lusty joy of life with hate.' "

The Crucial Issue: System-Ego or Person-Ego

That Jacobson still clings to the theory of innate instinctual aggression, in spite of having explained it as an object-relations phenomenon, appears when she writes of the growing child's "ambitious strivings to develop" and says, "Under the influence of his instinctual conflicts these strivings soon become highly charged with aggressive energy, and find increasing expression in competitive struggles with admired, powerful love objects, in particular with his rivals." [40] The facts of the child's immaturity and lack of relative mental and physical equality with his rivals, and his resulting insecurity, is enough to explain the tendency for aggression to emerge. Childhood, being the most vulnerable and dependent age, is most open to the arousal of fears more acute than any that we normally feel as adults. It is important to get our theory of aggression right, because so many avant garde writers are quick to make use of the idea that aggression is an innate biological instinct that ought to be expressed, and that one must be aggressive to be free and mature. Jacobson's view is that the *whole* of the original undifferentiated energy becomes differentiated after birth into *only two main drives*, libidinal and aggressive, which are radically opposed thereafter and either fuse or overpower each other. Thus these two energies must be *neutralized* by some hypothetical process, to make any other kind of energy available to the energyless structural ego, a purely speculative hypothesis, behind which lie the assumptions of the old classical psychobiology of instinct-entities operating outside the ego. The ghost of Rapaport's battle of the Titans in the unconscious still haunts and hinders the development of a truly clinical object-relations theory. Once we accept that the psyche-soma remains basically a unified whole whose fundamental energy is libidinal, and that aggressive drives develop in the service of the libidinal ego, we can take for granted that the whole-person ego retains its primary psychosomatic energy for use in whatever ways and directions are necessitated by its object-relations situation.

139

NOTES

1. Heinz Hartmann, *Ego Psychology and the Problem of Adaptation*, trans. David Rapaport (London: The Hogarth Press, 1959; New York: International Universities Press, 1964), p. 28.
2. *Ibid.*
3. *Ibid.*, p. 3.
4. *Ibid.*, p. 8.
5. *Ibid.*, p. 7.
6. *Ibid.*, p. 27.
7. *Ibid.*, pp. 30–32.
8. *Ibid.*, p. 32.
9. Donald W. Winnicott, *The Family and Individual Development* (New York: Basic Books, 1965), p. 3.
10. *Ibid.*
11. *Ibid.*, p. 15.
12. *Ibid.*
13. Donald W. Winnicott, "The Capacity to Be Alone," *The Maturational Process and the Facilitating Environment*, The International Psycho-Analytical Library (London: The Hogarth Press; New York: International Universities Press, 1965 *b*): 129.
14. *Ibid.*, pp. 30–31.
15. Donald W. Winnicott, "The Location of Cultural Experience," *International Journal of Psychoanalysis*, vol. 48, pt. 3 (1967).
16. *Ibid.*
17. *Ibid.*
18. *Ibid.*
19. *Ibid.*
20. Edith Jacobson, *The Self and the Object World*, The International Psycho-Analytical Library, vol. 67 (New York: International Universities Press, 1964; London: The Hogarth Press, 1965), p. xii.
21. *Ibid.*, p. 6.
22. *Ibid.*, p. 22.
23. *Ibid.*, p. 7.
24. *Ibid.*, p. 15.
25. *Ibid.*, p. 13.
26. *Ibid.*, pp. 15–16.
27. *Ibid.*, p. 15.
28. Sigmund Freud, "A Metapsychological Supplement to the Theory of Dreams," *Collected Papers*, vol. 4 (London: The Hogarth Press; New York: Basic Books, 1959), p. 140.
29. *Ibid.*, p. 12.
30. *Ibid.*, pp. 13–14.
31. Ernest Jones, "The Concept of a Normal Mind," *Papers on Psychoanalysis* (Boston: Beacon Press, 1961), p. 210.

32. *Ibid.*
33. *Ibid.*, p. 213.
34. *Ibid.*, p. 125.
35. Jacobson, *Self and Object World*, p. 11.
36. *Ibid.*, p. 10.
37. Bernard Apfelbaum, "On Ego Psychology: A Critique," *International Journal of Psychoanalysis*, 47, no. 4 (1966): 452.
38. Anthony Storr, *Human Aggression* (New York: Atheneum, 1968).
39. *The Yorkshire Post*, Leeds, England.
40. Jacobson, *Self and Object World*, pp. 49–50.

PART

II

Therapy

Chapter 6

THE SCHIZOID
PROBLEM

≡

Our consideration of theoretical developments in psychodynamic research has led us back, in the final chapter through a
reconsideration of the problem of aggression, into the midst
of the practical difficulties that human beings find in their actual day-to-day living in their human environment. The human environment into which the baby is born and in which
he or she grows up, through a series of fairly well-defined
stages, to adulthood and the hoped for goal of maturity of
personality, is infinitely variable. A sufficient number of babies
encounter good enough mothering, as Winnicott states, to enable them to emerge into their later social setting with sufficient stability and responsibility to "make a go" of living.
Nevertheless, our highly increased social awareness in this
century, both begetting and begotten by the growth of the social sciences, makes us unavoidably aware of how many in-
dividuals are unable to make this grade at all, and become
criminals, delinquents, psychopaths, cynical exploiters of their
fellow men, or else the opposite, lay-abouts, hippies living in
a fantasy world, drug-addicts, alcoholics, and so on. At one

time, those who did not fit into the social norms were either tolerated as interesting eccentrics, or simply condemned and punished for breaking the moral and social laws. Today we are able to see deeper into these problems, and although at varying points other people in society have a right to be protected against injury, we can make an understanding approach to the disturbing individual. After all, human beings are not born criminals or alcoholics. We are asking the question, "What has happened to this person to make him what he has now become, and what can we do about it?"

The difficulty of making stable and constructive relationships with other people, and playing a positive part in living, is not confined to the extreme cases mentioned. We have to consider two other groups, the emotionally ill (I do not use the term "neurotic" because it may too easily become a term of criticism or abuse), and those who are disturbed within the range of the "normal." As far back as 1908, when Freud was thinking solely in terms of his instinct-theory, he gave us three possibilities: we could "let rip" with our instincts and become criminal, or repress them and become neurotic, or "sublimate" them and become socialized, although this last course had somewhat uncertain and varying success. Today we would not state the problem in those terms, but there is an essential truth here. Instead of instincts today we would think in terms of an adult struggling with deep-seated unresolved conflicts and tensions in his personality that are a legacy from an unsatisfactory early life. The antisocial types are those who deal with their inner problems by simply working them off on other people, with the inevitable result that, whatever happens to them externally, internally their problems are never solved and they never become truly happier people.

On the other hand, those who do their utmost to prevent their internal tensions from simply breaking out on other people in hurtful ways are then forced to suffer a progressive increase in internal strife. They become divided against themselves until they break down into some kind of nervous illness to which a diagnostic label may be attached and for which they may be treated, perhaps by psychiatric drugs, or more constructively by trained psychotherapy, in which room may be found for the support of useful psychiatric drugs where that seems indicated. But those who become recognizably ill are not a class apart. When we come to examine closely all the variations of type and reaction among those who are considered normal and socially well adjusted, it is clear that very many of them suffer in only lesser degrees than those who become specifically ill, and from the same kind of problems. Our various types of trained social workers today are quite familiar with the problems of having to help "normal" people with their difficulties in maintaining good human relationships, whether in the handling of their children, or of their friendships, or marital or business relations, and with the varied fluctuations of mood that they suffer as a result of these problems. In short, we have now arrived at the time when it is apparent that man's major problem is not how to understand and master his universal physical environment but to understand himself and find out how we can help one another to live truly self- and other-fulfilling lives.

A Broad Clinical Picture Of The Schizoid Problem

Perhaps the major discovery of research into personality problems in this century is some understanding of the fact that "personality disturbances" can be grouped on two levels, one less serious and the other more serious. In stark textbook terms, these are psychoneurosis and psychosis, but we no longer think of those in the crude old ways as nerves and madness. We can see a continuum of causes in the course of any individual's development that can lead to these results. Although I do not think that Winnicott would dispute that in psychosis there can be, certainly in some cases, a hereditary or constitutional factor, which is very far from being understood, he sees reason in many other cases to reformulate the distinction in terms of two different groups of problem patients: (1) those who can be assumed to have had good-enough mothering and for whom serious stresses and strains in family and personal relationships later on in childhood and early adult life disturbed their proper development in these later phases of personality-growth. Whether or not we call their problems neurosis is of little moment. They struggle with the kind of difficulties *in* human relationships that experienced treatment can have a good deal of success in helping them to grow out of. They do not suffer any fundamental incapacity to make or enter into human relationships, and (2) those who cannot be assumed to have had good-enough mothering from the start and whose difficulties are far more deeply rooted. This group is not by any means simply to be identified with psychosis, even though psychotics who can be psychodynamically understood belong to it. They are the people who have deep-seated doubts about the reality and viability of their very "self," who are ultimately found to be suffering from varying degrees of depersonalization, unreality, the dread feeling of "not belonging," of being fundamentally isolated and out of touch with their world. This is broadly "the schizoid problem," the problem of those who feel cut off, apart, different, unable to become involved in any real relationships. Sometimes the so-called neurotic problems prove to be really of later origin and are not too difficult to clear up, but sometimes they prove to be defenses against the emergence of this deeper and more devastating experience of inner isolation. The problem here is not relations to other people but whether one is or has a self. I have no doubt that we are here faced with the most profound problem in human life, which we have already explored in theory, that of how a human being develops out of his original total infantile dependence and helplessness a sense of becoming a secure, inwardly stable self, strong enough to stand up against the external pressures of life in adult years.

With people in whom the solid foundations of secure and confident selfhood have been well and truly laid in infancy and early childhood, it is astonishing to how great an extent they can stand most abnormal pressures in adult years. We can recall how people have survived the horrors of political persecution, of concentration and prisoner of war camps, and have come through with their personality scarred and strained but intact, whole and able to start life afresh with constructive vigor. No less impressive are those less heroic cases of people who have stood the strains of family illness, economic misfortune, blighted hopes, and the bereavements and accidents that none can be immune from, and yet have survived with unbroken spirit, and especially without embitterment. Facts of this kind have forced us to look more closely at those apparently psychoneurotic problems held to be caused by upsets in later years, especially when they do not yield fairly readily to solution by what may be called the classical psychoanalytic approach. In fact it is now apparent that these problems in human relationships very often arise out of deeper problems of the inadequate development of what Winnicott called basic ego-relatedness, than is at first apparent. When that is lacking, the unfortunate individual's whole life is a struggle by all kinds of superficial relationships, techniques of dealing with people and events, and role-playing, to manufacture the feeling of being a genuine person. We cannot assume that the built-in experience of basic ego-relatedness is beyond damage. In our time we have to consider how far the extreme pressures of totalitarian political regimes backed by physical violence can push the strongest beyond their breaking-point. In a paper on "Alienation and the Individual," Pearl King discusses the way the "alienation experience in the individual," in the form of "passivity, anonymity, abandonment of individual identity was, in fact, one of the most important mechanisms of adaptation and defence which made survival possible" when the individual was utterly at the mercy of totally brutal and destructive terror-organizations.[1] Nevertheless, there were those whose personality survived, and we do not, for most practical purposes, have to consider such extreme cases. The person who becomes a depersonalized automaton under averagely normal social conditions is extremely ill, but lesser degrees of alienation, of disorientation and loss of healthy rapport with the human environment as a result of cultural displacement are a growing concern for sociologists and social workers, as Pearl King's paper shows.

The psychodynamic researcher must go to the ultimate roots of the problem, although considering all of the later stages; personality growth and ego consolidation begin, as Winnicott says, "at the beginning," with birth into the infant-mother relationship. Thereafter it proceeds through wider child-parent, scholar-teacher, employee-employer, and marital relationships, and often needs to lead on into the patient-therapist relationship, if a psychotherapist can be found. Many kinds of professional workers abound who will in various ways operate on the individual in difficulty, often in the interests of getting him to conform to the social norms and not be a nuisance. But more and more the psychodynamic outlook is permeating social work, and here we are only interested in helping the individual with emotional and personality problems to find and be his own natural, spontaneous, creative, and friendly self. Thus in turning to the problems of psychotherapy and treatment, I shall confine myself, in the interests of brevity, to what I believe to be the fundamental problem, the hidden hard core of trouble and illness, the schizoid problem. It is not a fixed entity, but as a matter of degree of uncertainty about the basic reality and viability of the central core of selfhood in the person, it can usually be found emerging sooner or later from behind everything else that has to be gone into.

Let us first consider a broad clinical picture of the schizoid condition. Schizoid, from the Greek *schizo*—"to split," is used loosely for both *withdrawn* and for more specifically *split* personalities. *Withdrawn* generally describes the introvert, quiet, shy, uncommunicative, detached, shut-in person. He may show *emotion* in a shy, nervous, shrinking, embarrassed way, or be *unemotional*, cold, aloof, unmoved, untouched by what is going on around him. The emotionally withdrawn person in fact feels strong needs and anxieties but is afraid of people and is retiring. The cold type is likely to make mainly intellectual contacts. When we consider the alternative term, "split personality," these differences are seen to be superficial. If the outer defenses of the cold, unemotional, intellectual are penetrated, he reveals a secret, vulnerable, very needy, fear-ridden infantile self, showing up in his dream and fantasy world, though split off from the surface self, the false self (Winnicott) that the outer world sees. The shy, nervous, reserved but needy and dependent person reveals under analysis a deeply hidden inner heart of the self entirely cut off from all communication with the outer world; shut in in an ultimate way as if regressed into a psychic womb in the unconscious, so that when they do find someone to depend on, they cannot feel or get in mental touch with them. The cold intellectual who hides an emotionally needy fantasying self also reveals deeper still this lost core of the personality. The profoundest ego-split concerns the existence of this lost center of a superficially organized self, leaving the person with no conscious capacity to love, to feel understanding, warmth, and personal concern for others but only being aware of a dreadful sense of isolation and nonentity within. One of the most disturbing experiences in psychotherapy is to lead a patient through the analysis of symptoms, Oedipal and other conflicts,

...stic, guilt-ridden and depressed conditions and ., hungry and hysterically clamorous needs for love, ,y to find himself becoming terrified by the emergence of an utterly intolerable feeling of total isolation. One patient, a grandmother, was outwardly cool and calm, and everybody admired her because she would not panic in a crisis, although this was actually because all outward show of feeling was secretly paralyzed by fear, and she reacted as an automaton. She had suffered from a series of psychosomatic and conversion symptoms for years. In a long analysis she lost all of these physical disturbances and then began regularly to start each session by saying, "You've gone miles away from me." I would answer, "You are mentally withdrawn from me." Then one morning she woke early, in the dark and in a panic, feeling she was blind, deaf, and dumb, completely out of touch with her world. Soon after that she said in a session, "I can't get in touch with you. If you can't get in touch with me, I'm lost." She then produced a dream which is the perfect description of the ultimate schizoid problem. "I opened a locked steel drawer and inside was a tiny naked baby with wide open expressionless eyes, staring at nothing." This is the one clearly defined psychopathological "entity" or experience to which the term "schizoid problem" could refer. It led me to propose, and Fairbairn to accept, the existence of a last final split in the ego as a whole, which I called the regressed ego, a part of the infantile libidinal ego in which the infant found his world so intolerable that the sensitive heart of him fled into himself. Winnicott refers to the "true self" of the infant, in an unnourishing environment, being "put into cold storage with a secret hope of rebirth" into a better environment later on, while a "false self on a conformity basis" is developed on the conscious surface. This gives the clearest meaning to the term "ego-splitting", although this is only the most serious example of it, as in the case of the young scientist who announced, "I am a non-person. I am a good scientist but I can't make any relationships with other people."

Apart from this extreme type of case, which, however, I believe in some minor degree at least is practically universal, the term "schizoid" covers too wide a variety of conditions for simple definition. It is more useful to recognize this hard core of the schizoid mentality and then use the term to denote a psychopathological trend to be found mixed up with all sorts of other trends, psychosomatic and hysteric, obsessional and depressive, sexual and aggressive, anxious and so on; and to be particularly watched as the pointer to the taproot of all other conditions. It can vary from a transient reaction that comes and goes inside one session to an undermining persisting basic condition, the power and ramifications of which only emerge from behind many defenses during a long analysis. Thus a young wife under analysis for depression came for a session just before going away on holiday. She was silent, unresponsive, and mentally miles away. I said "You're just going on holiday and you're frightened because you are going to be out of reach of me for two weeks. You feel you've got to do without me, and so you've started to do that already before you need. You'll be all the more anxious on holiday if you cut yourself off from me like this now." Her withdrawnness disappeared almost as soon as it was interpreted, but this one experience was enough to point to the probability of a fairly serious schizoid element in her mentality beneath her depression. Some time later this was confirmed dramatically. Her loud-mouthed and domineering mother-in-law was coming to visit her, and she came to session just before going to the station to meet her. She was pale, silent, out of this world. I simply said, "You're afraid of your mother-in-law." She replied in a small, tense, nervous voice, "I'm going further and further away. I'm getting so far away, I fear I won't get back. Am I going mad?" I reassured her she was not, and this is one point at which I disagree with the purist who says you should never use reassurance in psychoanalysis. Mostly, of course, reassurance would simply smother what needs to be analyzed, but in this case I felt it would recall her attention to the real issue, not fear of madness but withdrawal through fear of her mother-in-law. We must use common sense and not be too theory-ridden. I then encouraged her to talk freely about her feelings for this mother-in-law, and by the end of the session she felt more able to face her. Nevertheless, she had to telephone me to keep in touch for the next three evenings, but before the mother-in-law's return, she had become quite able to cope with her and not withdraw.

This example shows specifically that the schizoid reaction is a fear-product. The patient had had a near psychotic mother who had committed suicide, and a seriously neglected childhood. Her depression was partly guilt-feelings because of her bad temper and quarrelsomeness, but that itself was her fight to keep in touch with people despite her disturbed and withdrawn state of mind. One of my reasons for dealing so fully with the question of aggression, is that unless we see it clearly, we fail to see beyond it. A patient who said, "I'd rather hate you than love you. It's safer" was really implying, "I'm terrified that I won't be able to do either; that I'll feel nothing." Behind this patient's depression was a feeling of apathy, of the futility of life, which Fairbairn pointed out schizoid people often describe as "depression." She achieved a "cure" in seven years of not very intensive analysis, two sessions a week, which were reduced to one session a week during the last two years. Her illness had begun with the birth of her baby and her discovery that she had no feeling for her and no interest in her. This was diagnosed as "depression," a diagnostic label that psychiatrists nowadays appear to use as denoting a quite specific psychopathological entity curable with certainty and the appropriate drug. In practice, patients who experience widely differing states of mind all describe themselves as "depressed," and I have yet to come across a case where anti-depressant drugs have done more than shelve the patient's problem for an uncertain period of time. The birth of this patient's baby revived in her all of her pent-up feelings about her own deprived childhood, which gave plenty of cause for her feeling "depressed." For all practical purposes she has now maintained her freedom from depression for five years. Her analysis had dealt as much with her withdrawnness as with her depression, and she became able to "feel" for her baby, and to feel more enjoyment for life in general. She was able to stabilize at that point, and I made no attempt to probe more deeply into the regressed schizoid core that the history of her own infancy led me to suspect was probably there. It is dangerous to be a perfectionist, especially in dealing with the schizoid factor, the emergence of which can be devastating. Patients differ in their innate resources for recovery and for containment of what is unresolved. For all practical purposes the end of an analysis is wherever the patient can retain adequate gains and stabilize in terms of coping with and enjoying his day-to-day existence.

Relation Of The Schizoid Problem To Hysteria

Fairbairn was one of the first analysts to observe that severe hysteria has roots in schizophrenia. It would be more accurate now to say in the schizoid condition, which plays so large a part in schizophrenia when it is a truly psychodynamic problem. The usually psychiatric view of hysterics is that they are a nuisance, attention-seeking, demanding and overly dependent, manipulating other people including their physician, by an exhibitionistic use of their illness to command sympathy and help. They become experts in exploiting the secondary gains of illness. This type seems to be far removed from the cold, detached schizoid intellectual who poses as self-sufficient. This description of the hysteric, although it has its truth, is highly motivated by the doctor's defense against a very needy patient. The favorite prescription is, "Pull yourself together and think more about other people." It is true hysterics can exhaust and wear out the people they live with, but this situation, like that of manipulating the doctor, is complicated by the hysteric's anger at not being understood as having a genuine problem. The fatuousness of the advice is clear when we look into the real nature of the problem of hysteria. With obsessional and depressed people, the problem may be described in terms of the Freudian superego, or Fairbairn's antilibidinal ego being rampant, persecuting the grossly needy infant in the unconscious. Such patients are manifestly turned against themselves and are forced to deny their own needs. The hysteric condition is, at least on the surface, the opposite of that. The libidinally frustrated love-starved child who is terrified of being alone, is fighting for what after all is his elementary right to the primary supportive relationship that can alone enable him to live. If he had had it at the right time in infancy, he would not now be so cruelly undermined and dependent on other people. The hysteric is a neglected physically grown-up child, regarded as selfish by other adults because he cannot behave like an adult. He cannot because emotionally he is not adult. Genuine panic never lies far off for the severe hysteric because, desperately as he needs a supportive personal relationship, he is not really capable of believing in it and accepting it even when it is there to have. The most obvious reason is that hysterics usually do feel very guilty about their demandingness, and their superego punishes them severely in most painful conversion symptoms. One patient said, "I lose all my friends. I demand so much of them that they can't stand me." The sadistic superego, which is on top in the obsessional and depressed person, is very active underneath in the hysteric, attacking him in often almost intolerable physical pains. Hysterics feel guilty about their demandingness, not because it seems aggressive but because it seems weak and childish. The grandmother who had the dream of the baby in the steel drawer went through a marked hysterical phase in which she dreamed, "I had my husband and daughters and six guests to look after, and I just could not cope because I had a hungry baby under my apron clamouring to be fed." No wonder that her stable and long-suffering husband at times lost patience with her, only to make her feel all the more lonely and rejected. She would say, "I can't bring out my baby self to my husband. Though he's so good, he doesn't really understand. I've just got to be adult." But in fact she just could not, beyond a certain point. What was she to do? One hysteric patient, who did turn out ultimately to be schizophrenic, said, "I want to go back home and go to bed and be a baby and force my parents to bring me up all over again from the start." This grandmother could not do that literally, so she was driven to do it under disguise and pay a high price of suffering for it. She developed an acute pain in her right arm that made her helpless. Her doctor, who was convinced that there was something seriously wrong, sent her to a consultant, had X-rays taken, gave her drugs and two months of physiotherapy, but nothing did any good. She was too exhausted and distressed to travel to sessions, and both husband and wife felt desperate. Several days he was unable to go to work and leave her alone. I did what I rarely do. I went to see her at home, and after we had talked for a while, I pointed out to her that she was nursing her arm like a baby, and reminded her of her dream of the hungry baby under her apron who would not let her get on with looking after her family. She admitted that that idea had already occurred to her but she had dismissed it as being fanciful. However, she resumed her sessions, and in the next few weeks the acute pain died away. It was long after that, that the depth of her problem was shown by the dream of the baby in the steel drawer. She had had a seriously unloved

infancy and childhood. Her mother, who was of a higher social class, found that she had married a drunken sailor who
deserted her, and she was quite unable to cope with motherhood in that situation. My patient was the one who suffered
most, being the last and least-wanted child. Hysterics usually
make themselves as well as other people pay, by their demands,
for the hurts done to them, but they must hold on for their
very life because deeper than their guilt about feeling weak,
is their terror at their schizoid isolation, their actual inability
to enter into a genuine relationship even when they have the
chance.

One extremely ill hysteric middle-aged wife had a long
analysis before her schizoid problem developed clearly. The
eldest daughter of a pub-and-club-going father, with a mother
who was repeatedly pregnant and often ill, she was unwanted
at birth and at the age of eight years had to become the over-
burdened "little mother" to the family. She grew up to be an
introverted child who coped mechanically. After marrying a
much older good father-figure, she broke down when she had
her own baby. The baby grew up to hate the mother, who
was too undermined to mother her properly. For a long time
her analysis was occupied with working through the fears,
strains, resentments, jealousies, and guilts of both adult and
early childhood life, along with her angry longing for her
father's love and her destructive possessiveness and overdependence on her husband. In one dream she burned the whole
house of her childhood down with all the family in it, and
then filled with guilt, she rushed in and saved two favorite
children and devoted the rest of her life to them. Here was
revealed any amount of hate, guilt, and depression. But gradually and inevitably, deeper material from the schizoid level
began to push through. She began to exhibit the typical conflict between the need and the fear of human relationship, in
transference to her husband and to me, leading to the typical

schizoid in and out behavior, at one time responsive, at another resistant, aggressive, or aloof. She had two dreams in which she was a little girl standing trembling with fear at the door of a room in which I was sitting. She thought, "If I could get to him, I'd be safe," and she began to run to me. But in both dreams another girl of the same age (another aspect of herself) strode up and pushed her away, in the second dream hitting her cruelly in the face, just where she often suffered acute neuralgia pains. These are the dreams of a woman often criticized for her overdependence and demandingness. Because of this deep fear and inability to accept any real dependence on me, her inner sense of isolation began to be evoked, and she became subject to sudden panics, and feeling totally alone, cut off from everything. The schizoid core of her make-up emerged. So terrifying was this sense of utter isolation that once, when it broke through in the night, she panicked so badly that she swallowed all of her sleeping pills and her life was just barely saved. After that, when she found that my attitude toward her had not changed (she had expected me to be angry), she made steady progress until once more this horrifying sense of isolation began to develop. She pleaded for electric shock treatment, saying she really could not stand the sheer mental suffering. Since psychotherapy could not relieve this quickly enough, I had to accede to her urgent demand, and after E.C.T. she became profoundly regressed for about three months, a problem that was admirably managed by her husband. Once more she progressed slowly but demanded medication to protect her against that undermining sense of isolation especially in the night. We had to agree since there were times when she had to be left alone in the house. But I arranged that on one morning in the week, when her husband could manage it, she should take no pills at all and he would bring her over to me instead. She would arrive feeling very ill and by the end of the session would feel much calmer and in possession of herself. Gradually she became convinced that a person is better than a pill as a defense against the dread of isolation.

Therapy And The Need And Fear Of Relationship

This type of problem, the therapeutic support and mothering of a basically weak ego, is so utterly different from the therapeutic analysis of Oedipal conflicts over rivalries and jealousies, resentments and guilts in personal relationships, that Winnicott divided therapy into two kinds or levels: Classical Analysis for Oedipal problems, and Management for those who did not have good enough mothering at the start. The previous patient's mother used to go to work and leave her in the baby carriage for neighbors to watch her. It seems to me that one feels a more genuine rapport with truly depressed patients than with more basically schizoid people. It is all a matter of degree. It is not a question of the patient being either depressed or schizoid, as if they were mutually exclusive diagnostic entities, but to what extent depressed and to what extent schizoid. Whichever condition is stronger in the patient's make-up, the other one can be developed as a defense, so that, as Melanie Klein pointed out, patients can oscillate between the two. One fairly reliable criterion is that if a patient is more genuinely depressed, when he is angry he is more human and emotional; one can feel with him even if, in a negative transference, his anger is turned against oneself. When the schizoid patient is aggressive, the hate is cold, destructive, paranoid, and unfeeling. The depressed person gets honestly and bluntly in a rage, and then it is all over and he feels guilty at having hurt someone. The schizoid person can be implacable because he is unfeeling and can have a fiendish ability to find the weak spot and get under one's skin, and you feel that the aggressiveness is not over but lingers plotting under the surface. This is because the schizoid person is so essentially humanly isolated because his or her warmth of human feeling has never been evoked at the start of life. Because of this Melanie Klein linked closely the schizoid and paranoid states of mind.

Naturally not all schizoid people develop this cold sinister hate. Some human beings are more constitutionally easy-going and others more thrustful. The latter become aggressive more easily; the former take to flight. One gentle-natured female patient had grown up more afraid of a stern but certainly not violent father than there was real cause to be. Her mother, however, had a nervous breakdown when she was born and gave her a very uncertain start in life, and thereafter was by turns moralistically disciplinarian and emotionally possessive. The sensitive heart of this child shrank into herself, and she felt always alone but unable to venture out into human contacts. She dreamed once of seeing a couple kiss and she fled and hid in a small dark outhouse. Later she dreamed that she was inside a large metal ball with a small opening at the top, desperately trying to scramble up the sides and get out. I was outside and encouraging her, and at last she just made it. She felt a sufficiently real relationship with me for her isolated, secret schizoid self to be drawn out and rescued. But now, instead of feeling afraid of losing her ego in an emptiness, she felt the opposite fear of being overwhelmed and robbed of her own personality in a relationship. She dreamed that she was in a closed room with all of her valuable possessions and I broke in and was robbing her of them. Doubtlessly she was afraid of sexual intercourse and marriage, but there is far more than masked sexual symbolism in that dream. It means that basically that she did not feel strong enough to withstand any close relationship and maintain a viable personality *vis-à-vis* any other human being. The schizoid person conspicuously can neither do with nor do without the human relationships he or she needs.

The Late Development Of Schizoid Theory

The fundamental cause of the development of a schizoid condition is the experience of isolation resulting from the loss of mental rapport with the mother, at a time when the mother is the baby's sole environment and whole world, so that he has no alternative defense. The mother is the primary source of psychosensuous security, and the giver of the first relationship that can counteract the separation-trauma of birth. Only in this subjective experience of quickly and reliably restored security, can the ego-potential of the infant psyche begin to develop. It is sometimes said that Oedipal and depressive problems are problems of instinct-control, whereas schizoid problems concern relationships. Thus Fairbairn, describing how he first became aware of the deeper schizoid problem, cited a patient who said, "You're always saying I want this or that instinct satisfied, but what I want is a father." But this did not go far enough and he later came to see that the ultimate want is for the mother, because without her the infant psyche has no means of getting a start in becoming a personal ego. If we are to say that psychoneurotic disturbances concern relationships with other people, then we shall say that the schizoid condition concerns a relationship with one's self. It constantly emerges in the form of chronic uncertainty as to whether the patient is or has a self, owing to feelings of emptiness, nonentity, and dereliction. So often it turns out that it is because the patient has no well-assured sense of his own selfhood that he is unable to make satisfactory relationships with other people. We have seen how the schizoid problem obtrudes in the hysteric, but it comes out just as plainly in the paranoid, depressed, obsessional, phobic, and other types.

We must now place the schizoid problem in its theoretical context. The phenomena were always there, but their distinctive importance was only slowly realized. Freud distinguished between transference neuroses and psychoses, and held that psychoanalysis was only relevant to the neuroses because they permitted transference relations to be formed, which he regarded as impossible in psychosis. We can now see that this was the first step toward recognizing that the problem of those conditions that go deeper than neurosis is that they make personal relationships, and therefore transference, extremely difficult if not impossible, because there is no adequate self or ego with which to make a relationship. Analyzable psychotic and borderline cases highlight the schizoid problem, but it is there in psychoneurosis as well. Jacobson writes:

The rising interest in the problem of identity is probably caused by the widening scope of psychoanalysis and the growing number of borderline or even psychotic patients who call on the psychoanalyst for help. In such patients we can observe processes of regression that lead to a grave deterioration of object-relations and of super-ego and ego function, with dissolution of those essential identifications on which the experience of our personal identity is founded.[2]

I take this to be a recognition of the emergence of the schizoid problem.

Another way of expressing this was to say that to be suitable for psychoanalysis, a patient had to have an intact ego, implying that the trouble in psychotic, borderline, and other cases more deeply disturbed than neurosis is the lack of a proper ego. That is true enough, but what is an intact ego? Is there such a thing? In practice the term is meaningless, but it was many years before it became clear that the problem of the ego, not of instincts, is the one radical problem throughout the whole gamut of mental illness. Intact ego could only describe a whole and healthy personality. Freud and Breuer began with hysteria as a psychoneurosis. In the 1890s they could not have known that it went back into schizoid and schizophrenic problems. They were dealing with conversion symptoms, florid exhibitionistic reactions (the notorious *arc du cercle* symptom seems to have died out; I have seen only one patient in thirty years who came very near to producing it). The hysteric's intense sense of unmet need, clinging and dependent like a little child and liable to develop into transference sexual problems, scared Breuer off. Freud had the courage to go on. It was this early concentration on hysteria that caused Freud to place so much stress on sex. Broadly, sexual phenomena express needs for supporting personal relationships, when they are anything more than a purely biological appetite, "a bit of physiology" as Winnicott once stated it. Fairbairn regarded sexual symptoms, whether of over- or under-intensity, as hysteric conversion phenomena, the substitution of a body-state for an ego- or personality-state.

By contrast, aggression expresses anger at deprivation of needs, and when turned back against the self, it generates the guilt and depression that led Freud on to his next phase, the investigation of obsessional neurosis, the superego concept and eventually the development of structural theory. It was both fortunate and unfortunate that Freud began with hysteria; fortunate because it compelled him to be the first man ever to make a serious, truly objective, scientific, and radical investigation of sex. This urgently needed to be done, because until it was done, the phenomena of psychoneurosis remained hidden behind a smoke screen of sentiment, morality and pseudomorality, and physical symptomatology that was not recognized as being of psychic origin. So thoroughly did he do this job that the clinical facts were established once and for all. It was only his initial explanatory hypotheses that needed to be revised. On the other hand it was unfortunate that Freud had to be so preoccupied with sex at the outset, because it led him to overestimate its importance. Sexual phenomena, which were in fact symptoms of deeper disturbances, were long regarded as the primary causes of human troubles. Sadism and masochism were written up as instincts, sex and aggression were confused and wrongly related, and sexual libido was regarded as the entire life-drive. Freud's critics, who accused him of pansexualism, although not technically correct, had more justification than was admitted. Nevertheless infantile sexuality, sexual (sensuous) tension in other than genital areas; oral, anal, and peripheral (skin) libidinal excitations; the mixing of sex and hate; sexual symbolism in dreams, myths, and art; guilt over sex in the unconscious, and sexual involvements of children and parents, all this was established for the first time in a scientific way. This was a tremendous achievement. Freud simply accepted a sex instinct and went on with his research.

One thing at that stage was not clearly recognized, that people can have sexual reactions that appear to be normal and are physiologically uninhibited, and yet be incapable of loving, of genuinely feeling for another person in a deeper and more personal way: that in fact sexual activity is frequently resorted to as a substitute for loving when that is lacking. Genital sexuality was mistakenly equated with personal maturity. It was not clearly seen that though maturity includes sexual potency, the opposite is not true; sexual potency does not by any means include personal maturity. It was not seen at that stage that satisfactory sexual functioning does not depend on the existence of an instinct, but on sex appetite being a part of, and expressing the over-all purposes of a whole mature ego or self. Freud missed that, largely because no satisfactory concept of the person existed at that time. He was led on clinically from problems of sex to problems of control, from needs to aggressions and guilts, and from hysteria to obsessional or compulsion neurosis. This was as necessary a stage of investigation as was sex and hysteria. Freud could not have gotten much further with the study of hysteria on the basis of simple instinct theory. That only permitted theories of the fate of impulses, gratification, frustration, control, revolt, guilt, and punishment. Freud's classic psychoanalytical phase was a biosocial theory of morality. Hence Rieff's description of him as a moralist. The opening up of sex problems led to the equally factual investigation of moral phenomena and the psychic development of conscience, the superego theory, and the all-important fact that conscience can be pyschopathological. The analysis of superego operations in illness was based not on biology but on internalized personal, parental relationships.

This led Freud to the great divide in his theory, greater than he himself realized; the shift of emphasis from instincts to the centrality of the ego took place from 1920 onward. Not until interest moved beyond the control of separate id-drives or instinctive impulses and centered on the ego, the whole person, the self relating to the object-world, was it possible for the schizoid problem to begin to emerge; for it is the problem of there being a self. Before then, the schizoid state was treated largely as a constitutional problem. As late as 1944, in *Psychoanalysis Today*, Kardiner does not mention the schizoid underlay in hysteria, and Hinsie treats schizoidism as a constitutional factor in his chapter on Schizophrenia. But once we start with the ego as a whole self, the point of view changes. Depression could still be treated as guilt over bad impulses of aggression hurtful to loved-objects, but the schizoid state of withdrawal, detachment, and flight from reality, is clearly an ego-problem, a self in the grip of fear and isolation. But total flight would mean death, so the infant has to find out how both to fight and flee at the same time, and ego-splitting is the inevitable result. With part of himself he holds on to the hostile outer world, in either an aggressive, or demanding and dependent, or even an emotionally aloof intellectual manner on the level of consciousness; while with a deeper part of himself, his sensitive feeling capacity, he takes flight, and withdraws into himself. The live core of his psychic being becomes the baby in the steel drawer, Winnicott's "true self in cold storage." Thus one very able professional male patient dreamed that he lived in the bottom of a dugout, covered by a steel turret with two periscopes for eyes, two holes for tape-recording incoming sounds, and one hole for broadcasting his messages. He appeared calm and unmoved to other people; in himself he felt like a frightened child cowering down inside his dugout. His turret was his depersonalized head dealing with the outer world. His major symptom was severe chest pains when he went out walking, which faded away as he returned home (to his dugout), a conversion hysteria symptom.

Hysteria, The Embodied Self And Ego-Splitting

Hysteria symptoms are more common than frankly obsessional ones, and serious obsessional symptoms are so formidable a problem because the patient has been driven to despise and persecute the needy child within, which the hysteric is so much more aware of. Fairbairn suggested the slogan Back to Hysteria, so let us look once more at hysteric sexuality. Obsessional neuroses, with the elaborate use they make of compulsive thinking and ideas, clearly derive from, or make use of, later phases of development. The hysteric in his conversion symptoms is on the very primitive level at which, in the baby's experience, he is one sensuous body-mind whole. His brain is not yet developed enough for a mental fantasy life to operate, although it will soon begin to do so, and lead on from images to ideas. The earlier the disturbance therefore, the more likely it is to manifest itself as bodily suffering, and thus the more likely it is that both need and suffering will run into sexual channels. Fairbairn maintained that sex, like any other function, is only one area in which personality problems may be worked out, but the earlier and the less sophisticated the level on which the disturbance is experienced, the more likely it is that the symptoms will be sexual. The particular problems expressed along the channel of sex will clearly be the most basic ones, the infant's need of love in the form described by one patient as "the comfort and security of the contact of warm flesh," the sense of being in relationship that is given by the bodily mothering and handling that Spitz and Sullivan stressed, with the accompaniment of emotional warmth in giving and receiving. This is, in itself, something quite distinct from genital sexuality, and it seems to me that we ought consistently to distinguish between them by using two terms, sensuous and sexual. However, in the course of growing up, *the needs for sensuous comfort and security that are basic in the hysteric easily exploit the genital and specifically sexual channel.* Any strongly felt bodily need can always flow over into the excitation of the organic sexual apparatus, so that even a very tiny male infant can have an erection of the penis. In the analysis of hysteric symptoms, I believe it is important to help the patient to understand that *physical sexual symptoms mask a more broadly based and significant need for "personal relationship" in its basic security-giving value, which began as a need for the nursing mother.*

In the more specifically genital sense, hysteric sexuality oscillates between overstimulation and inhibition. Overstimulation reveals the infant's hungry and angry demand, and shows its schizoid basis most horrifyingly in the male psychopath who rapes and murders a little girl. To such a degree of dehumanization can the total frustration of basic human needs reduce a human being. But, apart from the extreme paranoid psychopath, sadistic impulses set up reactions of fear, guilt, and horror, and instead of uncontrolled sadism we find masochism, sadism turned against the self, and the inhibition of direct sexuality, and the hysteric suffers in his own body, as conversion symptoms, something of the torture he might otherwise inflict on someone else. It is just as inhuman and schizoid to torture oneself. All of this frustrated, torturing, and tortured sexual hunger and primary emotional need is basically infantile, a legacy of gross environmental failure at the start of life. Fairbairn wrote, "Hysteric genitality is so oral." A female patient said, "I want something in my mouth and something between my legs all at the same time." One pale, silent, aloof woman woke in terror one night feeling she was nothing but a big mouth ready to devour everyone, and dreamed of standing with a vacuum cleaner and sucking into it everyone who went by. In intercourse she dared not have an orgasm until her husband withdrew because she felt she would somehow bite off his penis. She said, "I daren't love. It's all devouring and being devoured."

This overwhelming neediness, resulting in a schizoid flight from human relations can only be understood not as failure of satisfaction of a sexual instinct but as a total withdrawal reaction by a hopelessly deprived love-starved ego. The tragedy is that although the schizoid so desperately needs human relationship, he cannot enter into it because his fears do not allow him either to trust or to love, and he feels so weak that he expects the mental proximity of another person to overwhelm him. He may oscillate between being in and out of personal relations. When he is afraid of his inner loneliness, he may rush into a precipitate overintense friendship or infatuation, or try to substitute sexual activity for the personal relationship he cannot achieve, and end up disillusioned because he is still basically withdrawn. When his fear of commitment to close relationship is dominant, he will become shy, detached, asocial, or sexually anesthetic, frigid, impotent, and inhibited as a substitute for genuine independence and for the capacity for self-reliance of the nonanxious person. Sexual inhibition is more deeply psychopathological than overstimulation, because it is more totally dominated by schizoid withdrawal and despair. Neither are desirable, but at least in sexual overstimulation, the starved ego is putting up a fight for life, however dangerous the results, while in sexual inhibition something vital has gone dead, given up the struggle; fears have mastered and repressed needs. Both are conversion hysteria symptoms masking a schizoid problem. Either a starved infantile ego or else a frightened and withdrawn one finds expression through the body. In inhibitions, a lost function is a clue to a lost part of the self.

In all of these problems, we are faced with a human being who has lost psychic unity, who develops conflicting and incompatible reactions to his own needs and to the people and situations he meets. This is what we mean broadly by ego-splitting, and we need a terminology to express this inner disunity, not an instinct terminology but one that clarifies the strongly persisting differences of attitude and reaction within the over-all ego, which prevent it from presenting a united front to life and undermine self-confidence. Freud gave us a start with his structural scheme, id, ego, and superego, which represented mainly the problems of depression, guilt over bad impulses, both sexual and aggressive, and punishment. An aggressive superego, or primitive conscience representing identification with authoritarian parents, rouses guilt in the ego and represses instinctive drives in the id. This scheme, however, being tied to a very superficial concept of the ego, could not represent ego-splitting. The personality differentiates internally on the basis of good and bad experiences in object-relations. If early experience is good enough, it is "digested" to use Bion's term, and as Fairbairn said, it simply promotes good ego development, and abides as stable character and pleasant memory. If early experience is bad, the infant cannot cope with it, and it remains, to use Bion's term, as "undigested foreign bodies" in the psyche. The inner world of Melanie Klein comes into being. Internal bad objects can only be dealt with by repression, internal conflicts, or projection, and balanced by internal good objects if possible. In this structural pattern, all the individual's past life is built in and assimilated to the basic dynamic pattern formed in infancy. This complex structural pattern into which the ego differentiates persists through the years and becomes conscious in the fantasy life of dreams, symptoms, and transference relationships. It persists as a reinforcement of infantile weakness and the source of psychopathological breakdown. Only through the help of a good analyst can the patient outgrow the internal disharmony that his fantasy expresses, by working through transference relations and developing a steadily more integrated psychic structure through new good-object relations, and thus find his natural selfhood.

Melanie Klein provided most of the material but not the concepts for a new theory of endopsychic structure, nor could she do so since she retained the nonpsychological impersonal "id" for what is really the infant's primary natural self. Fairbairn dropped the term "id" and substituted the term "libidinal ego" to denote the pristine unitary but as yet undeveloped needy nature of the child. Libidinal ego seems to me to be the obvious psychoanalytical term to represent the infantile starting-point of our psychic life, and it makes possible the conceptualizing of subsequent development, either as growth in ego-strength, or else as ego-splitting and the proliferation of ego-weakness. The internal bad objects are at first the exciting but frustrating and unsatisfying aspects of parents, on the primitive paranoid level generating the images of sheer persecutors, and on the later depressive level, moral accusers. Freud fused and confused these two aspects in the term "sadistic superego." Fairbairn's term, "antilibidinal ego" exactly describes the "against all natural needs" attitudes of the internalized authoritarian parents. What confuses and disturbs the infant is that bad parents excite his needs (if only by being there and being his parents) and then fail or refuse to satisfy them. He is faced with both exciting and rejecting or denying internal bad objects, and his weak ego splits under the strain. He in part identifies with the rejective parents, develops an antilibidinal ego and becomes a self-hater; but in part he goes on being excited and having his needs stimulated, and goes on being a libidinal ego fighting for his rights.

But deeper than all this, if the struggle is too hard, a more secret split-off part of himself withdraws from the hopeless struggle, and becomes a lost regressed or withdrawn schizoid ego. All of this is hidden on the conscious level by a conformist central ego avoiding trouble by idealizing parents in real life, often in the most unreal way, as when a seriously ill hysteric young woman announced in her first session that she had the most wonderful mother on earth. By this means she avoided admitting to herself how much fierce hate of her mother she secretly harbored inside. Fairbairn's terms for the basic threefold pattern of ego-splitting, libidinal ego, antilibidinal ego, and central ego (to which I would add the schizoid regressed or withdrawn ego) is a development from Freud's first experimental definition of endopsychic structure, but has the advantage of being more accurate because it is based on later developments in research. It is the most convenient way I have found for summarizing our present state of knowledge of the internal disunities caused by an overly disturbed development in the earliest years. Here, in this complex pattern of ego-splitting or loss of primary psychic unity, with all the weakness and internal conflict it involves, is the root cause of personality disorders in later life; and the most vulnerable part of the self is the most hidden part, the schizoid ego, cut off from all human relationships in the depths of the unconscious. To reach and help this lost heart of the personal self is the profoundest problem posed for psychotherapy.

NOTES

1. Pearl King, "Alienation and the Individual," *British Journal of So-cial Clinical Psychology* 7 (1968): 81-92.
2. Edith Jacobson, *The Self and the Object World,* The Interna-tional Psycho-Analytical Library, vol. 67 (International Universities Press; London: The Hogarth Press, 1965), p. xii.

Chapter 7

PSYCHOANALYSIS
AND PSYCHOTHERAPY

We cannot simply identify psychoanalysis and psychotherapy because there are nonanalytic forms of psychotherapy based on reassurance, supportive or authoritarian advice, hypnotic exploitation of infantile dependence, or some kind of supposedly therapeutic activity that some psychiatrists call the talking cure, none of which aim at the radical results that psychoanalytic treatment at least seeks to make available for the patient. I think no one would want to deny that some degree of help may be given by these other therapeutic methods, especially since some patients are either unwilling to accept or are unsuited for the more thoroughgoing analytical approach. Moreover, the more radical results that are the ultimate aim of psychoanalysis expose it to greater risks of failure; although even when the full results hoped for do not materalize, it is far from true that nothing has been achieved. Some patients decide to terminate treatment before the analyst feels they have gained all they could from it, but it is for the patient to decide and he can always return to analysis again later, as not infrequently happens. Analysis makes no promises, but offers to the patient a reliable and understanding relationship for as long as he wants to use it, to explore his personality problems in depth and free himself to develop a more natural and spontaneous self. An experimental psychologist, Max Hammerton of Cambridge, recently said in a B.B.C. broadcast, "I am happy to stand confidently by my assertion that, so far, there is no evidence that Freudian therapy has ever cured anybody of anything." [1] His "happiness" about this was very obvious from his whole talk, and analysts are handicapped by not being able to publish so much material that is so entirely private and confidential. In any case, Hammerton safeguarded himself by asserting that "particular case histories, however dramatic, prove nothing by themselves," and that he would only accept "a statistical comparison of experimental and controls groups." Under certain circumstances this could be possible, and an extremely thorough example of such an experiment carried out by over two hundred research workers from the University of Wisconsin and the Mendota State Hospital, over a period of five years, with encouraging results, is recorded in "The Therapeutic Relationship and Its Impact: A Study of Psychotherapy with Schizophrenics," edited by Carl Rogers. It is all the more important that this was not carried out specifically by psychoanalysts, for it suppports what is, after all, the fundamental assumption on which psychoanalytic treatment rests, namely that a reliable and insight-promoting personal relationship can be therapeutic. The critics of psychoanalytic therapy usually ignore the implication of their views, which is simply that persons *qua* persons, who can and do so obviously influence each other for ill, cannot influence each other for good; a conclusion that would nullify all that is most important in parenthood, friendship, and marriage, let alone psychoanalysis.

But there is a further difficulty about Hammerton's physical-science method of proof: so very often a psychoanalytical success is registered in a case that is so utterly individual and unique that no possibility would exist in practice of finding an adequate parallel case to serve as a control. Many years ago a patient was referred to me for depression. He had also suffered for years from chronic recurring severe sinusitis, which was never cleared up without medical and even surgical treatment, always to flare up again later. In the course of analysis, he began to delve into his extremely unhappy early life and the fact emerged that he was left alone to nurse his mother on her deathbed. It had always puzzled him that his memory of her last day was a total blank. Then he developed another severe bout of infected sinuses, and literally rushed into my room at the next session, and blurted out the following: "Last night I woke up and the whole forgotten memory of mother's death burst into consciousness. She went mad at the end and died cursing me. It was too horrible. I blotted out the memory of it, but as it came back to me, my sinuses just opened and the pus poured out, and this morning my sinusitis has gone, for the first time without medical help." Moreover, it has not recurred. This certainly is an unusual case, and qualifies for Hammerton's "however dramatic," but he would have difficulty either finding a comparable control case or ascribing the cure to anything other than the psychoanalytical opening up of what had been repressed and unconscious. Such a case points out a fact that we must never ignore, that in psychoanalysis science is for the first time challenged to understand and thereby explain the unique individual, and that this must lead to a new development in our concept of what is science. Bronowski in *The Identity of Man* says that there are two kinds of knowledge, knowledge of the machine that is science, and knowledge of the self that he ascribes to literature. He regards knowledge of the self, however, as just as genuinely "knowledge" as is knowledge of the machine. Psychoanalysis claims that it must be possible to have a science of knowledge of the self as well as of the machine, but it will not use the same kinds of method or concept. It will be the science of psychodynamics, and must be free to evolve its own terminology to handle its own unique phenomena, those of our subjective experiences of ourselves and of one another as "persons in relationship." This science is in being and has grown out of the psychotherapeutic endeavor to help disturbed persons by going along with them in tracing their problems to their personal origins in their emotional life history. The ultimate and permanent importance of Freud in the history of thought will rest on the fact that it was he alone, practically unaided, in the face of fierce prejudice and opposition, who laid the foundations of psychodynamic science and a psychotherapy based on it.

Fairbairn once remarked to me, "The more we study the psychology of the ego, the longer analyses become." That is certainly true. In fact, the cases that prove to be capable of fairly quick resolution are cleared up as quickly as they were in the early days of psychoanalysis. It is simply that the study of the ego has made us ever more aware of those factors that go far deeper into the individual's psychic make-up. Freud rightly at first restricted psychoanalysis to the treatment of the psychoneuroses and ruled out the psychoses because he regarded transference as impossible in such cases. That in itself is a demonstration of how entirely psychoanalytic treatment rests on the basis of personal relationship between analyst and patient. Where no such relationship was possible, Freud held analysis therapy to be inapplicable. It was thought that in neurotic and Oedipal problems the ego was intact and capable of making a relationship and was treatable. What Fairbairn was noting was that the ego psychology initiated by Freud himself was driving research ever deeper than the Oedipal and psychoneurotic problems, and that in many, if not all, cases these proved to be defenses against something fundamental that concerned, not so much the existence of disturbed personal relationships as the possession of a fundamental core of selfhood, an ego real enough to be capable of relating at all. What at first set the limits of psychoanalysis for Freud has turned into the very problem that it has now recognized as its major concern: the schizoid problem where the secret isolation of the heart of the patient's life, giving him a feeling of unreality and nonentity, makes transference the major problem rather than the criterion for treatment.

We need not spend time on the psychoanalytic therapy of the psychoneuroses. So much is known about that, that we can take it for granted. Anything I could say about it would only concern those cases where patients cling to their psychoneurotic conflicts and symptoms as a defense against being plunged into the deeper and more frightening experiences that have to do with their not being able to experience themselves as a proper self at all. I shall devote the remaining section to consider the treatment of these deeper problems about which classic psychoanalysis opened the way to understanding. We are thus dealing with cases of a more than usually disturbed kind, and this may find expression in disturbed behavior, although it also may find expression in, as it were, no behavior at all, the manifestation of a sense of helplessness and unreachableness. We may call these patients borderline cases if their active behavior poses a problem, or just schizoid if they are more than ordinarily aloof and unresponsive. The point is that they do not abide by the rules of classical psychoanalysis, whatever we may think these to be. The patient whose problems are genuinely psychoneurotic and no deeper, will usually, in spite of the resistance he may consciously or unconsciously feel, want to talk about himself and appreciates having a genuinely concerned listener who does not start criticizing or telling him what he ought to do. He will, if given the chance, free associate without being told in technical language that that is what he is doing. He will talk about something that is really emotionally worrying him and let it lead on, until a broad picture of his over-all situation begins to emerge. That is what happens in the easiest cases, and that is just is what is interfered with in proportion as his problems, instead of being cleared up, lead him into deeper and more disturbing depths. My impression is that psychoanalysts are no doubt thankful for a case of simple psychoneurosis, but they are more and more intrigued by and interested in those patients who present profounder problems. They compel us to ask questions about our methods of treatment.

Winnicott stated the problem simply and clearly when he said that psychoneurosis calls for classical analysis, but the inadequately mothered patient who has been disturbed from the beginning calls for management. Analysis in such cases, is, however, not ruled out or omitted. Whenever it proves feasible to do a bit of real analysis, it clarifies confused situations enormously, but one is forced to be thinking even more about the patient's basic needs than about his problems, or to be thinking about his problems all the time in the closest relationship to vital fundamental personality needs that have never been adequately met. The ultimate need is to feel sure of one's reality and viability as a person, the need to be. At this point I feel it is necessary to take a good look at the term "therapeutic," or "psychoanalytic *technique.*" I do not wish to create the impression that I want to challenge terms hallowed by long usage just for the sake of challenging them, but I think there is an important issue at stake in looking critically at both the term "psychoanalysis" and the term "technique." They are both products of the early days when Freud quite naturally took it for granted that if he was to create a *science* of the human personality, it must necessarily conform to the traditional methods and type of terminology with which his extensive physical science education had made him familiar. He could not foresee that he was breaking entirely new ground in venturing beyond knowledge of the machine into the problems of knowledge of the self, and that he was creating a new area of science in psychodynamics. The terms "analysis" and "technique" seem to me to belong properly to the methods of the physical sciences. The machine, whether it be an atom, a motor car, the human organism, a plant, or the solar system, requires, as it were, to be taken apart in thought, and its constituent parts identified and related, and their modes of interaction established. On the basis of this kind of knowledge, it becomes possible to put parts together and create a new machine. We cannot, however, deal with human personality in this way. I think an attempt to do it is the aim of all conditioning and behavior-patterning, but the result is not a live creative person but a social conformist, perhaps a good totalitarian party-man, or even a "typical business executive" or a "typical anybody," but not an original unique person with creative capacities to produce the unexpected. We cannot see persons as parts assembled into a reliably working whole whose behavior can be predicted. One of the early criticisms of psychoanalysis was that it broke people into pieces and did not put them together again, and some critics suggested that we needed a theory of psycho-synthesis. They did not see that they made the same mistake. You cannot understand a human being by an analysis of his parts, mechanisms, and so on, nor recreate him by a synthesis of those same parts. A person is a whole self and so unique that it is impossible to find, among all the millions of human beings that have existed and do exist, any two who are exactly alike. When a baby is born, he contains a core of uniqueness that has never existed before. The parents' responsibility is not to mold, shape, pattern, or condition him, but to support him in such a way that his precious hidden uniqueness shall be able to emerge and guide his whole development. This is a variable factor, stronger in some than in others. It needs the support of a social and cultural environment, but it is, in some, so powerful that it will burst through all the bonds that parental training, social usage, and educational pressures may inhibitingly load him with. One of the demands made by Hammerton is that a true science must enable us to predict! In fact, the more possible it is to predict consistently exactly what a human being will do, the less of a real person he has become, and the more he presents what Winnicott calls "the false self on a conformity basis." I can think of techniques for conditioning people to behave in prescribed ways, and I can think in terms of the analysis of the mechanics of their operation, but I cannot think in terms of a technique for setting a person free from his fears so that he can discover his own unique individuality. I cannot think of psychotherapy as a technique but only as the provision of the possibility of a genuine, reliable, understanding, and respecting, caring personal relationship in which a human being whose true self has been crushed by the manipulative techniques of those who only wanted to make him "not be a nuisance" to them, can begin at last to feel his own true feelings, and think his own spontaneous thoughts, and find himself to be real.

I think of a patient who said: "There is a dream that I've often had for years. I know it so well, it's all familiar to me while I am dreaming it. I know it's the same dream that I'm always having, but as soon as I'm awake it's all gone, except that I know I've been dreaming that same dream again. All I can say about it is that I feel something has been stolen from me, I'm robbed, there isn't any real me." I could see more of her true potentialities than she could. When she came to pass through a time of severe crisis in her real life, and was afraid that she would break down under the strain, while we went as deeply as we could into all that came to light in dreams and other ways of the details of her reactions to it all, so that she could develop her own insight into how she was handling the situation (and we may, if we wish, call this analysis), I felt convinced that she would cope with the situation and come through a stronger person. As that began to happen, she said at one session, "I would have broken down but for you, if I'd had to face it alone. I've done that before when in difficulties.

But I sensed that you felt sure I would win through. Your faith in me enabled me to have faith in myself." This is not analytical therapy, it is personal relationship therapy. I did not use a technique. If I had tried to reassure her, or convince her, that could well have been called a technique. In fact, I simply saw in her something that was there, that her parents had never seen in her, and that she did not see in herself because all the personal relationships of her early life had done nothing to release her real whole self.

Terms such as "analysis" and "technique" are too impersonal. They remind me more of engineering than of personal relations. One can teach a technique, but cannot teach anyone how to be a therapeutic person. The point of the training analysis is not to teach theory or technique but to free the real person in the candidate. One can teach negatives, such as you must not reassure, criticize, moralize, give advice, laugh at (though you may laugh with), or interrogate the patient. You can teach that it is wrong to try to force premature interpretations. It has always been taught that the right time to interpret is the moment when the patient is nearly seeing something important and just needs a bit of help over the last bit of resistance. But you cannot teach a candidate how to know when that moment has come. That will depend upon his sensitivity and intuitive understanding, and they are expressions of his maturity and reality as a human being. Until I feel I have come to know a patient fairly well, I often suggest a possible interpretation, which he may follow up or discard. "Do you think that what you are talking about might imply this or that?" If I ask myself what interpretations I make and why, I realize that only in the broadest sense are they based on what I have learned from the textbooks, and my theory is always under pressure from what is actually coming to me live from the patients' own struggles to say what they are going through. I find myself saying things to patients today that I realize would never even have occurred to me in my early days in therapy: and finding that they are right, that they set free something in the patient and he gets on. I can well remember my early days when I had only the textbooks to go by, and felt stuck when the patient did not oblige me with signs that his problem had been cleared up. Moreover, I do not think it is possible for us to put into a book all the insights we have gained by experience over the years. They are not written down in our minds, as it were, in conceptualized form. We do not know what insight we have until we are in the live situation with another human being presenting us with, not a problem to be solved, but an imprisoned self to be understood and freed. Our accumlated experience has made us the actual persons we are right now, and our intuitive understanding of the patient comes, not out of what we intellectually know but out of our capacity to relate, to feel for and with this particular person, in the same way as Winnicott says that the mother "knows" her baby in a way that the trained doctor, nurse, and psychologist cannot know him. Nevertheless, it is out of the major, salient aspect of our immediate, on-the-spot insight into patients that we gradually distill out some clear concepts that go into our theory of human nature, as psychodynamics.

In the same way, I do not instruct a patient to lie on the couch. I wait to see what he will do, and when and why he wants to do something different. The whole matter was put to me quite clearly by one patient. He stood in the middle of the room and looked around, and then said, "I'll feel too grown up if I sit in that arm chair, but I'll feel too like a baby if I lie on that couch." In fact for a long time, he sat sideways on the couch. Then he sat up in the chair and his therapy became much more difficult and sticky. It was a defense, and he gave it up and went back to sitting sideways on the couch. Then one session he half turned around and put one leg up on the couch, and at the next session he put both legs up, and then when he really relaxed lying on the couch, accepting the dependent, helpless, anxious infant he actually felt to be, then things really began to move, and truly therapeutic results began to accrue. The point I am making is that one cannot practice a stereotyped technique on patients: one can only be a real person for and with the patient. I am sure that this is why so much effort is put into trying to find impersonal scientific techniques, or pills or what not that will make some kind of difference to the patient that he will accept as a cure. It is a far more exacting thing having to be a real person for another human being, so that he can come to feel at last free to be his own real self. In the course of this, we shall make use of everything that we have learned from our own analysis, and from the textbooks and journals, but only in the way in which we have assimilated it into our very make-up as persons who are able to be just what is needed by the patient who may say, "I can't reach you. If you can't reach me I'm lost." This is what the more schizoid patients are always saying to us one way or another. "I haven't got a real self to relate with. I'm not a real person. I need you to find me in some way that enables me to find you." Only then is the really schizoid patient rescued from his profound internal isolation, and linked up, as a mother links up her baby as soon as he has been thrust forth into the great empty world, and creates for him the first and most important, if as yet very dim, experience of relationship.

There are, of course, times when the only therapeutic way of relating is not to relate, when the patient would feel smothered or overwhelmed or swallowed up, or else persecuted and paranoid. In a relationship, one must know how to wait. Freud's early recognition of the fact that the possibility of treating psychoneuroses by psychoanalysis depended on the fact that the neurotic is capable of transference, that is, of personally relating with real feeling to the other person who is immediately there, was a profound insight. Before any wider application of psychoanalysis could be attempted, it was necessary to fully explore all the problems in personal relationships that were experienced by patients who were sufficiently real as persons to be capable of relating, even if their ways of doing it were disturbed by emotions that belonged to their childhood relations with quite other people. This is considered classic analysis. When we have a patient who only needs help at that level, the problem of making a relationship as such hardly arises. The therapist finds that the patient relates to him fairly directly, even if at times it is in a hostile way, in a negative transference. I think this is why for a long time the essentially *personal* nature of the psychotherapeutic relationships was obscured by the more obviously analytical nature of what went on in the relationship. It is with the ever deeper explorations of ego-psychology that we have been thrust up against the much more fundamental problems of those who do not feel sufficiently real as persons to be able to make a relationship. But we cannot now do what Freud, at first, had to do, simply say that this problem lies outside the scope of psychoanalysis. As Jacobson says, more and more borderline, schizoid, and even psychotic patients turn to analysts for help. Though success in these cases is much harder to achieve, yet certainly patients as seriously ill as this have proved to be capable of being helped, and in the process have compelled analysts such as Winnicott to recognize that here they must be more than mere analysts. Classic psychoanalysis of ambivalent human relationships, if it has any success in such cases, only removes conflicts that were being maintained as defenses. The result then is that the patient's true problem, the extent of his inner isolation and unreality, can emerge with frightening intensity.

Interpretation may still need to be the therapist's most visible mode of relating to the patient, but it will not be interpretation of Oedipal conflicts. It is more likely to take the form of having to get the patient to see that whatever activity he engages in, he is driven to do it in a tense, compulsive, anxious way because he really feels he has got to fight to keep himself alive at all, to struggle to convince himself from moment to moment that he really is a somebody. He has to prove himself to himself all the time. He is so often therefore unable to relax, and dares not go to sleep, and may actually consciously feel and say, "If I go to sleep, I fear I may never wake up again." Such patients will dream of falling into a bottomless abyss, and fears of dying are very real to them. Their reaction to real-life responsibility is to drive themselves frantically in an effort to cope as long as they can keep it up, and to then succumb to an overmastering need to escape by either a mental withdrawal or an apparent physical breakdown into exhaustion. With one such case Winnicott installed an expert nurse with instructions to nurse the patient as if she were a helpless acute pneumonia case, and himself did her shopping for food. This shows how starkly and simply the deepest root of illness in a schizoid patient may prove in the end to be a catastrophic lack of sheer mothering, which somehow the therapist has to understand and find out how to remedy. In Winnicott's case the result was a success. I shall illustrate this by the dream of a male patient who related that he was with his mother in the house where he was a boy. It seemed dilapidated and unhomely. His mother went out and left him, and later he felt hungry and went out to search for her. At last he found her with a group of friends chatting and eating in a restaurant. He said, "What will I do for meals," and she only stared at him and said nothing. Dejectedly he went back to the empty house, and as he went in he was suddenly terrified to find himself faced with a huge Alsatian dog that grabbed him in its mouth. Here, if you wish, is a clear example of oral masochism, of hate, of angry hunger for the mother who failed him as he turned back against himself. But that analysis does not go far enough. What was the alternative to feeling this fierce uprush of rage? At least the struggle to contain and cope with it inside himself did something to enable him to feel he was still in being. Behind that, and as its only alternative, there lay nothing but the empty house, which was an experience of the collapse of his childhood ego in a world empty of mothering. Thus at one vital point he did actually fall into an early childhood illness, lying listless and seemingly dying on his mother's lap, and the doctor could find no physical reason for his condition. He was saved by his mother's sending him away from herself to a motherly relation who had children of her own and knew what a little child needs. When material of this kind emerges in treatment, it is relationship not analysis that is required, although it is still necessary to help the adult in the patient to understand what is going on, and we may call this analysis if we please. It is not analysis in classical terms. It is not Oedipal analysis. The mother in this case is not a sexual love-object for possession of whom the child feels rivalry with the father. The mother is the other essential person in the earliest pre-Oedipal two-person relationship. It is in this relationship alone that the baby can get a stable start in feeling to be an ego, a person, and his sense of reality will depend at first entirely on the reality of the mother's relationship to him. In classic Oedipal analyses the importance of a therapeutic relationship is not absent. It is merely not so conspicuous because the patient's need for it is not as great. With schizoid, borderline, and some psychotic patients, this need can emerge with imperative force and dominate the treatment, and it is only its emergence and acceptance by the therapist that makes a good result possible. In fact, at every level, analytical interpretation is simply the medium of an understanding relationship. In the *British Journal of Medical Psychology*, Yvonne Blake of South Africa describes how she treated a criminal psychopath, how his aggression was disarmed when he discovered that she really understood him and was on his side, and how he passed through a period of acute fear of madness into a phase of profound dependency, after which he emerged with a growing personality of his own and ended treatment as a constructive member of society.

However, this problem of the extreme dependency of the more seriously ill patient is far from being a straightforward problem to handle. The more schizoid the patient is, the greater degree of dependency he basically feels, and the harder it is for the patient himself to admit it and accept it, and trust his most vulnerable, isolated, potentially true self to the therapist. At times he fears and dreads a real relationship even more than he needs to. It was the meeting with this kind of resistance that I was referring to when I said that there are times when the only way of relating to the patient is not to relate, to be still, quiet, saying nothing, and if he begins to be disturbed by what at last he may feel is lack of interest, find the best way of interpreting this as respect for his need not to be interfered with, or imposed on, or mentally invaded, or have something put across on him. As it dawns on him that the therapist really understands and respects his fear of being helped against his will as it were, this may be the beginning of that all-important ingredient in all true relationships, a capacity to trust another person who can be seen to be trustworthy. Even then he may fear his demands will exhaust the therapist. It is really for reasons of this kind that therapeutic enthusiasm has always been recognized by analysts to be a dangerous thing, arising not out of true care for the patient, but out of the therapist's need to be supported by successes.

One of the most difficult problems in the treatment of the patient with a basically weakened ego is that he is not only much more dependent on his therapist, once he can accept it, than the psychoneurotic patient is, but also he is much more vulnerable to and at the mercy of his outer world. This is most true for his immediate family life and his work, but at times can even extend to his being more than normally disturbed by the world situation. Most normal people today know what realistic anxiety is in relation to international events, and it would not be a sign of maturity to feel nothing at all about Vietnam, an Israel-Arab war, or the Russian-Czechoslovakian situation. I have found, although not invariably so, that the psychoneurotic patient can be so occupied with the immediate problems of his day-to-day relations with the people important to him, that he may not spare much mental energy for the consideration of world affairs. On the other hand, the patient with the basically weakened ego is terrified of the whole external world, and may become abnormally anxious that every crisis will precipitate an atomic war. With one such patient, real improvement became visible when he ceased to panic in advance about every possibility of international trouble.

A much more serious problem, however, is the chronic vulnerability of such patients to the pressures of everyday real life responsibilities, with which they never feel equal to coping. Moreover, it so usually happens that they are bogged down in very strained relationships with those they live with, who have not been able to understand their illness and cannot stand the strain it imposes on the family. In one such case, a very ill wife was undoubtedly the cause of her husband's thrombosis, and had been so unable to mother her child adequately that she definitely provoked hostile relationships by her angry demands. Such a family is likely to drift from crisis to crisis, and just as one thinks some real improvement could begin to be stabilized, some domestic explosion completely undermines the patient again. In some cases the patient is too ill to be managed at home and has to be hospitalized. I have been fortunate in having the cooperation of a hospital superintendent who made it possible for me to carry on psychotherapy with those few patients who, for a time, had to become inpatients. This has worked well. In other cases, where a good result has been obtained, after a long treatment, I have always felt that the patient owed as much to those he or she lived with, as to me. Without a stable and supportive family basis, I do not think it is possible to treat some patients with any success. Where psychotherapy must go deeper than impulse-conflict and deal with the basic condition of the ego or self whose impulses they are, the overriding factor is that a real self, a whole-person-ego, can only grow in so far as the patient can be drawn into a basic security-giving personal relationship, at first with the therapist, but also, and with his help, with other members of the family. At the deepest level, psychotherapy is replacement therapy, providing for the patient what the mother failed to provide at the beginning of life. The biggest problem is that the patient, never having had such a security-giving relationship, has no deep feeling for it, and cannot really believe in it. The problem of psychotherapy may then be put as Fairbairn has stated; how we can get inside the patient's inner world as a closed system, in order to get a process of natural fear-free growth of personality started? This is a problem that may well daunt us and seem to be insoluble. I do not pretend to have any slick answer. I can only say that in some cases I have failed, but in some other cases I have had such clear-cut success as to leave me in no doubt that this therapeutic process of regrowth of personality from the foundations is a real possibility, not with every patient but certainly with some. One very important factor is the patient's own determination not to be satisfied with anything else.

An example of such a case is relevant at this point. I give it, not because I think it is a possible practical aim for all patients. Clearly it is not. For psychiatrists under pressure from such heavy case loads, it is simply out of the question. Most analysts will only be able to carry a few such cases. I present it because the fact that such a result proved possible at all has the most important implications for the nature of human personality and for the true ultimate goal of psychotherapy. The patient, a spinster who came for treatment in the late thirties, was socially very isolated, always changing jobs and lodgings, obsessed with fixed irrational hates of a variety of somewhat irrelevant things, and a quite ferocious attitude of self-depreciation. She was given to outbursts of rage over trivial matters, which she always turned against herself in the form of physically punching herself, and despising herself. Her mother, a superficial and completely self-centered woman, had not wanted any children and hated the only child she had, and used to beat her on any provocation. The child identified with her mother, and continued for years to treat herself in the same way that her mother did. She frequently had nightmares of being persecuted by her mother, sometimes in person, sometimes in symbolic form, as when she dreamed of being pursued wherever she went by a vulture who was constantly pecking at her. Many of the details of her case material could be explained in classic analytical terms, as when she dreamed that she had married her father and they were just going to bed when her mother burst into the room in a rage and dragged her away. However, orthodox analysis of such material made little difference, other than clearing the way for the emergence of her basic problem, a deep feeling of utter fear and weakness that she felt she dared not give in to. She hated bed and sleep, saying, "When you are asleep you are just not anybody." She lived an extremely strenuous life, and seemed physically strong. After a number of years of analytic therapy, she began to recognize and admit a real dependence on me, and began to grow listless, and tired after the day's work, and ailing. In panic, she rushed back to resistance, aggressiveness, and strenuousness, and recovered her physical energy and hardiness. But slow changes were going on over a period of more than ten years of analysis, and she refused to give up, saying that if this treatment failed, there was no hope for her. Gradually she returned to the admission of her dependence on me, and her recognition of how deeply she felt to be a total nonentity in her self. Her defensive identification with her persecutory mother slowly waned, and she became the persecuted child, and as before, her physical health deteriorated badly. The ways in which she went on living with her mother in her dream world showed signs of a changing situation. Then, after about fifteen years of analysis, in one session she fell quiet for a long time and then looked up and said, "It's safe now. She's gone. It's the turning point. I'm going to get better." That was over two years ago, and the recuperative process was complex and needed to be understood as we went along. In her worst periods of disturbance she had been accustomed to scream, "I'm not a woman, I'm a man, a man." Now it emerged that for her, being a man meant being strong enough to master her mother, and being a woman for her meant being weak, being the terrified little girl she had been all her childhood. Now that her mother had faded out of her mental make-up, she accepted her femininity quite happily, but continued to feel physically weak and had in fact become bodily frail. She realized that it was an automatic assumption with her that she could only be bodily weak if she remained happy now to be a female. From that time, this conviction gradually lost its hold on her, and her health and vigor improved. The companion she lived with said, "It's a pleasure to live with you now. You've changed completely." The change has become so stabilized that she has now ended her treatment, and is simply a normal, contented, friendly person, and has had promotions in her work. Naturally, in such an instance the criticism that "case histories, however dramatic, prove nothing" carries no conviction at all with me. We are dealing here with a different order of reality, which cannot be dealt with by orthodox traditional scientific methods. The one indisputable fact is that this woman's illness always focused on the hold that a persecutory mother had on her unconscious mental make-up (the mother having been dead many years), and that it cleared up from the moment this hold was undermined. The only factors that had any bearing on its undermining were (1) our constant investigation of its manifold effects on her life, both conscious and in her deeper emotional dreaming self, and (2) the new sense of basic security she experienced from the fact that she could replace her mother by my reliable understanding and the supportive affection steadily shown to her by her companion. That what we are and can be as persons is bound up completely with the quality of our most important personal relationships should be so obvious as to need no proof. If what is sought is not simply the removal of symptoms but a qualitative change in personality in the direction of greater internal self-confidence, stability, and maturity, not only *freedom from* fears, but *freedom to* enjoy life in a natural spontaneous way, with the ability to use whatever gifts one has creatively, then the only truly therapeutic factor is that of good personal relationships that combines caring with accurate understanding. It has been suggested to me that there is no protocol, in the sense of a formal statement of the transaction, for Fairbairn's object-relations theory as applied to treatment. Fairbairn himself would certainly not have tried, or wanted to try, to set out any such formal statement of what might be called an object-relations technique of psychoanalysis. My own view is that there is and should be no such thing. I regard object-relational thinking as the gradual emergence to the forefront of what was always, from the beginning, the real heart of Freud's revolutionary approach to the mental illnesses he was faced with; that is to say mental disturbances that are not specifically the result of physical causes, but profound disturbances of the normal courses of emotional development of human beings as persons. That psychotherapy is simply the application of the fundamental importance of personal relationships, in the sense of using good relationships to undo the harm done by bad ones, follows automatically.

The specifically psychoanalytical aspect of this kind of psychotherapy is really a part of the content of a good therapeutic relationship carried far enough. It involves both the capacity to understand the patient and the capacity to communicate that understanding in such a way that the patient can accept it. The experience of being understood comes as a tremendous new vitalizing factor to some basically lonely people who feel they have never understood themselves, and that no one else has understood them. Suddenly they realize that they are no longer alone in life. It is here that our need to build up a psychodynamic theory, constantly tested in clinical experience, arises; for if every patient is ultimately unique in his individuality, it is also true that every patient shares in our basic constitutional heritage as human beings. All human beings have fundamental things in common. We can come across the same kinds of conflict, of emotional disturbance, of defensive symptomatology, in patient after patient, even though in each separate patient these have an individual nuance. We can pool and sift our knowledge of these experiences so that we can obtain a constantly corrected and expanded body of information about the common stages of human development and how these can be disturbed and distorted. But we can only apply this to any given individual under the guidance of our own intuitive understanding of what is going on at this moment in this patient. Psychoanalysis has, now I believe, uncovered the deepest and most awe-inspiring problem from which human beings can suffer; the secret core of total schizoid isolation. A recent suicide was reported to have left a tape-recorded message, "There comes a time when you feel there is no meaning in life, and there is no point in going on with it." Far more people than we know have this feeling deep within them, although not all to the same degree of intensity. We may well pause before this problem, which no psychiatric or behavior therapy technique, or classic Oedipal analysis can solve. The only cure for an ultimate sense of isolation and therefore meaninglessness in life, in anybody, is that someone should be able to get him back into a relationship that will give life some point again. Can we be sure the patient can stand its being uncovered, or dare we leave him alone with it lest it break out willy-nilly and destroy him? Can the patient be sure that we can stand it and support him until a new trust and a new meaning in life begins to be born again in him? One cannot always know the answer to these questions, but where patient and therapist are prepared to stick it out together, then, at the risk of tragic failure, a profoundly rewarding success can, in my experience, in a significant number of cases be achieved. I do not know how this can be statistically validated by the hard pressed general practitioner of analytic therapy, but the patient knows when he is literally "born again."

NOTES

1. Max Hammerton, *The Listener* (August 29, 1968).
2. Yvonne Blake, "Psychotherapy with the More Disturbed Patient," *British Journal of Medical Psychology* 41, no. 2 (1968): 199.

INDEX